WOMEN ON THE COUCH

AN ANALYSIS OF FEMALE PSYCHOPATHOLOGY

Also by Cláudia Bernhardt Pacheco:

- *Healing Through Consciousness — Theomania: The Cause of Stress*

Co-author in the books:

- *From Sigmund Freud to Viktor E. Frankl: Integral Psychoanalysis*
- *The Technique of Interiorization*
- *The Decay of the American People (and of the United States)*
- *Liberation of the People — The Pathology of Power*
- *Öppna Ditt Fönster (Open Your Eyes)*
- *Psicoterapias Alienantes*

CLÁUDIA BERNHARDT PACHECO, Ph. D.

WOMEN ON THE COUCH

AN ANALYSIS OF FEMALE PSYCHOPATHOLOGY

PROTON PUBLISHING HOUSE, INC.
São Paulo • New York • London

Cover
Carlos Gomes de Freitas II

Translation and Revision
Margaret Pinckard Kowarick

Design & Typesetting
Trilogical Graphic Design, Inc.

ISBN — 0-939019-02-7

Library of Congress Catalog Card No.

Published by Proton Publishing House, Inc.
Av. Rebouças, 3819 • 05401 São Paulo, SP • Brazil
547 West 110th Street, 2nd floor • New York, NY 10025 • USA
6 Colville Road • London W11 2BP • England
Printed in Great Britain at The Bath Press, Avon

Table of Contents

Part I

A Study of Psychopathology

Part II

A Study of Sociopathology

Part III

A Study of Sanity

Closing Message

Dedication

I dedicate this book to all of the worthy women — past, present and future — who struggle to make truth, beauty and goodness prevail in the world, regardless of the cost or the pain it may cause.

I also dedicate this work to all of those honest women who, because they lack the correct orientation, are deluded, maltreated and confused, unaware of the real causes of their suffering and unable to resolve their problems.

Not least, I dedicate this study to all those worthy men who have sincerely tried to help us, men who have alleviated our suffering as best they could. Indeed, they deserve the best of partners, women capable of returning their love in like measure.

My work is the realization of a commitment I have with my Creator, who made it possible for me to liberate myself from the bonds that kept me from developing.

I would like to thank Dr. Norberto R. Keppe, my analyst and teacher, the person who patiently planted the seeds of awareness in the garden of my life and who can now see his efforts come into bloom.

Lastly, I want to thank my patients, who furnished most of the valuable material included here, and who accepted my help and trusted my orientation.

I offer this book to you, the reader, in the hope that we will soon see society become more humane, a society in which the woman fulfills her true role of manifesting, with dignity, love to all the world.

Cláudia B. Pacheco

An Explanation to the Reader

In this book I have tried to analyze in greater depth both the individual psychopathological causes and the sociopathological causes that underlie female suffering and problems. Not only do women suffer, they also cause offers to suffer. Often this is inadvertent due to alienation or lack of proper orientation, sometimes it stems from a response to strong social and educational pressures, or it may even be the result of envy and narcissistic attitudes of which the woman is unaware and thus cannot control.

Lately, women have been the object of frequent study by both the feminists themselves and by sociologists, psychologists and legal experts who try to decipher the question of why the position of women has been inferior and unequal to that of men in an overwhelming majority of cultures, past and present.

Having noted that much has been overlooked in regard to a more specific analysis of feminine psychopathology (psycho = *related to the psychological;* pathology = *the study of disease;* psychopathology = *the study of mental illness*), I have tried in this work to focus on all facets of the woman: her difficulties in relation to herself, to men, to the family and society, and to her Creator.

It is important that the reader realize that when I speak about women, although I seem to generalize, extending all of the concepts herein described to all women, in fact I refer mainly to those pathological attitudes which pertain to a greater or lesser degree to the feminine gender as a whole.

Obviously there are many women of great worth, and even those who are most unbalanced still always possess some measure of sanity.

The fact is that in science, which deals with experimentation, it is necessary to base ourselves on general, universal, fundamental principles and at the same time respect the individuality of each human being. Thus, in this study of women, the premise that each case is unique and must be analyzed separately holds true. In trilogical psychoanalysis this scientific rule is honored.

The most difficult undertaking I have ever attempted was this study of the psychopathology of women. Never before had I experienced such difficulty; never before had ideas become so tangled, nor had it ever been so arduous to organize my thoughts and put them down on paper. As the project developed, I felt an increasing resistence, a growing laziness. Other projects appeared to which I gave preference in order to avoid the task before me.

On the one hand I experienced a feeling of extreme sorrow as I verified the degree of insanity we women have reached; on the other, I saw that when a woman perceives her problems, she does, in fact, develop greatly and very rapidly.

I believe that I am going to have a great deal of difficulty in being heard, not only by the women themselves, but also by the many men who patronize and take advantage of female craziness, which today has become an institution. Many times in conversations and meetings, when I broached the question of women's problems, there were men who reacted ferociously in defense of females who were no more, no less than their "perfect mothers" — women who pampered and petted them, making them the "little kings" of the household. These men were far less willing than most of the women to accept my words.

When one woman listens to another, no matter how hard she may try to avoid it, she knows the truth when she hears it because within herself she feels when it is genuine. Men are different. They consider the ill intentions and intrigues of women as mere utterances, and only through their own experience in male-female relationships can they identify these as being true or false. This is why it is more difficult for men to accept a new female image.

Truly, I would like the women and men who read what I have written here — and who are shocked at first by certain feminine aspects I describe — to make an effort to consider these hypotheses with all seriousness. These concepts have, in fact, been applied on a large scale in dealing with the women I have had the opportunity to orient, and the results have been highly encouraging.

I have also been careful to enlist the help of other women, and of men as well, who are directly or indirectly involved in this new comprehension of the woman.

It is satisfying to note that women are gradually becoming aware of the fact that their situation in society is entirely abnormal. They are reacting, fighting for equal rights, searching for more direct participation in deciding the destiny of their own lives and the lives of others in their families.

Nevertheless, what worries me is that the underlying causes of the problem are not analyzed in their entirety. In other words, the question that has remained unanswered is why the woman has put herself — or, if you prefer, has allowed herself to remain — in such a chaotic position, a sub-human position, in the scenario of civilization?!

If we fail to analyze the causes of female subdevelopment dialectically; that is, if we focus solely on the social aspects of the problem, we will be making a grave mistake. Female psychopathology must be analyzed deeply if women are ever to deal maturely with their new responsibilies and their freedom.

That is why it was so difficult to write this book. All along the way I had to be extremely careful not to permit my own psychopathology to interfere in my analysis of the facts. Similar care was necessary in regard to the data used in the research, especially with female authors who in many cases tended to take more aggressive positions in relation to men and to other women as well.

Some of these authors erred by portraying women as innocent victims at the mercy of macho beasts. Others went to the extreme of criticizing their fellow sex savagely, in a show of envy and intolerance.

It is extremely difficult to be just, because the human being is not perfect enough to judge others or himself fairly. Nevertheless, what I will attempt to do here is analyze as objectively as possible those points which have gone unquestioned up to now or which have been considered taboo by society as a whole.

An Admonition from the Author

The reader will note that I use the terms God, the Creator, the devil and other similar words a number of times throughout the book. You may associate these with the censoring way of speaking that is typical of religious fanatics. Nevertheless, all of the facts discussed herein come solely from scientific experimentation.

I want to make it very clear that I speak strictly as a woman scientist, although I understand that the true science is trilogical science, which unifies philosophy, science and spirituality in order to treat the human being, with his feelings, thoughts and actions, in an integral manner — the only way, in fact, that modern man accepts being treated.

The understanding of God is not the same in science as it is in the religions. Although it has been our custom to deal with God in the churches, philosophy in the universities, and science in doctors' offices, from now on we should accustom ourselves to the unification of all aspects of human life, a unification that must guide the civilization of the Third Millennium.

Preface

The individual who begins to do something worthwhile in life, the person who makes up his mind to do something really good, begins to experience an extraordinary process of continually-expanding awareness.

A vast range of possibilities for realization begins to come into view. And the more such a person does, the more clearly he sees how much there is to be done and how many thousands of possibilities there are.

Nevertheless, in order to accomplish anything we must have a certain amount of past realization and learning as a foundation. That is why the person who truly begins to put himself into action (but not in work that enslaves or alienates), comes to realize how much he could have learned to do in the past but did not.

Yet such awareness of having wasted our lives in the past is also the starting point for building a strong foundation for the future. If we are to accomplish anything worthwhile, we must heed our consciousness of our past errors or ignorance and use this as a base. For example, if I should decide tomorrow to become an opera singer, when I begin to take singing lessons, it will soon become evident that I should have begun dedicating myself to the study of music a long time ago if I am to be able to sing even a few songs in a wobbly voice today. Awareness of time wasted in my life will press upon me relentlessly.

Many of us cannot bear such consciousness for very long. In fact, most of us choose to give up trying and promptly revert to a position or situation that alienates us, one in which we are not forced to see how much time we have squandered in our lives. The collective result of such behavior is that humanity in general is becoming increasingly superficial, increasingly shallow-minded.

The woman's situation has, in fact, become critical. Today, when one of us makes up her mind to free herself from inertia and accomplish something good, beautiful and true that nourishes the spirit and affords genuine pleasure (not pseudo-pleasure, like that of spending money, for example), an accomplishment that brings happiness and freedom, she discovers that there are an enormous number of restrictions and difficulties to be overcome. Some of these are obstacles of a social nature, others are economic or psychological.

Whichever they may be, a great deal of effort is necessary to surmount them, free oneself of inertia, and embark on the path to freedom of realization. Indeed, it will not be easy for us to create a reality in which we are no longer dependent and alienated, a reality in which we do work that is worthwhile and meaningful for humanity.

Greater still is the effort we are going to have to make to stand the discomfort and frustration we are bound to feel as we become aware of the extent of our past uselessness, of our incapacity, and of how we women have wasted our lives and thrown away our talents until now.

We are also going to have to transform the whole erroneous philosophy of life and the mistaken preconceptions that have been built up around the female. It will not be easy for us to begin to feel, think and act correctly.

Nevertheless, my friends, the effort will be well worth it!

Part I

A Study of Psychopathology

I will make you enemies of each other: you and the woman, your offspring and her offspring. It will crush your head and you will strike its heel.

Genesis 3:15

1

Envy, Inversion and Women

My readers will note that I use the word *envy* many times throughout the book. By envy I mean the attitude of destroying that which is good in one's own life and the life of others. Freud called this type of behavior the death instinct *(thanatos)*, which he believed came from a natural unconscious.

Freud noted, in fact, that in the most seriously ill mental patients (the psychotics) the pathological element of envy was highly pronounced. Later, Melanie Klein, likewise a noteworthy psychoanalyst, carried out still deeper study of the role of envy in unhealthy psychological processes. Finally, Norberto Keppe contributed an even broader understanding of envy, having verified that it is indeed the root of all human difficulties, in the individual psychological sense as well as the social sense.

The meaning of the word *envy* in Analytical Trilogy is different from the meaning commonly given to this term. Envy, as its Latin origin indicates *(invidere)*, means "not to see." Thus, by basing the true meaning of the word on its etymological origin, we conclude that an envious person is one who is unseeing, who does not want to see. What is it he is not willing to see? That which is good, beautiful and genuine — those things that are self-existent — for everything that exists in and of itself is good. Indeed, reality was originally only good, beautiful and true before the human being began to spoil it out of envy.

In Trilogy, we consider envy to be the basis of all psycho-pathological problems; that is, we believe that all psychopathic attitudes stem initially from envy and are directly linked to it. These destructive attitudes are: theomania (the wish to be god-like); megalomania (having grandiose ideas), a component of theomania;

narcissism (adoration of one's self, one's body, one's personality); arrogance (thinking oneself always right, a know-it-all attitude); alienation (lack of awareness of reality); and inversion of values, the most serious of all.

Inversion, a direct consequence of envy, refers to an inverted view of everything in life — an attitude that causes us to fear and reject the good things while respecting and desiring the bad. Our fear of loving, of being hurt or destroyed by love, is one example. We are, in fact, reluctant to be good, patient and dedicated because we are afraid that we will not receive due recognition and in some way will be harmed.

Instead, we prefer to believe that if we are rational and cold, carefully calculating the advantages and disadvantages of each step we take, we will be able to avoid the more serious risks. We think that if we keep ourselves from caring for others too deeply, we will avoid problems such as rejection, abandonment by the loved one, separation, ingratitude and the like. In anticipation of such consequences, we withdraw from everything and everyone we care for most. And we never lack reasons to justify our unwillingness to accept what is good in life, to enjoy life, to be relaxed and happy.

Thus, the envious person is the person who opposes, who says *no* to what deep inside he appreciates the most: all that is beautiful, all that is true. Nevertheless, the individual denies what is good without clearly realizing it. He may, in fact, steer his entire life in the direction of unhappiness, guided by this unperceived (inconscientized) pathological attitude.

Some refer to it as masochism, others call it sadism — the wish to suffer and make others suffer. We are constantly trying to spoil the good moments in our lives and the lives of others. And this attitude that we call envy is so strong, so infernal, that we are rarely able to free ourselves entirely of the habit.

Each of us justifies this universal envy with a system of ideas, a philosophy of life. Christianity and Judaism, for example, have long preached that we must suffer if we are to enter heaven (as though God wished us to suffer and, like an executioner, awaits the first opportunity to punish us).

No one is entirely without envy. However, one person may be more conscious of his envy than another and thus be able to discern to some degree the reasons for his bad choices in life.

This whole concept also applies, of course, to those powerful individuals who, out of hidden envy, prevent both the people and themselves from being happy. Indeed, they spoil their own lives, not only the lives of those they exploit.

I do not believe that God is pleased to see that although he created a paradise for us to enjoy, free of charge, with everything in abundance that we need to live a richly fulfilling life — happiness, health, contentment, joy, pleasure and realization; in short, the best of everything — we have allowed a small group of mentally ill people, who hold all of the power in their hands, to take from us that which is ours by right.

These are the people who have created wars, hunger, poverty, disease, destruction — a truly chaotic situation on the planet — and yet they still complain about life, all with our connivance.

We are living in a dialectical hell; that is, on the one hand, we have inherited from our forefathers a civilization based on a 'philosophy of problems,' a mistaken idea which, on the other hand, we continue to nourish and pass on to our descendants. Why not put a stop to this infernal cycle? The only ones to suffer would be Lucifer and those who are like him in their envy and desire to destroy.

The great majority of human problems have been created by the sickest people in society with our tacit consent, consent by omission. These problems are all out there, and the attempt to ignore our consciousness of them is not going to help in any way. Indeed, we are forced to recognize the fact that our intention has not really been to overcome our problems at all. The popular Brazilian saying: "Why simplify things if you can complicate them?" clearly illustrates the fact that we are unable to accept something good without spoiling it in some way.

The individual with power in his hands is an expert at creating complex and problematic social systems which invariably cause incredible difficulties for everyone. Many female power-wielders in the home are experts at creating problems in family life and in their own private lives in relationships with their children, friends, boyfriends, husbands, lovers, etc. People seem to have learned that life without problems is not life.

If you, the woman who is reading this, are just a tiny bit honest with yourself, you will recognize your attitude. How many times have you, in a good moment with your boyfriend, your husband, your children, or even alone with a beautiful sunset, for example, let your mind fill with ideas that elicit all sorts of worries — thoughts which inevitably disrupt your peace of mind and the peace of mind of the others around you?

Some women try to control this process to some extent and at least spare their loved ones by allowing them to preserve their peace of mind. Others are savagely envious, bent on creating chaos in their own lives and the lives of those around them.

A good example of inconscientized envy (envy not clearly perceived by the person himself) is my patient, Mrs. T.I., a woman over sixty who began psychoanalysis in an attempt to improve the quality of her life. With her children grown, some grandchildren already, there was little for her to do at home and she was beset by feelings of deep insatisfaction.

Totally dependent on her husband, financially, socially and psychologically, she sought some kind of constructive independence in which she could do something productive that would also provide another source of income for the family.

During the first two sessions of analysis, she made good progress in understanding her problems and the way to solve them. She became interested in reinitiating the artistic activities she had given up some years before, making fine quality handcrafted ceramic objects and tapestries.

By setting up her own Trilogical Enterprise, she would have the necessary freedom to do what she liked to do and at the same time have enough flexibility in her work schedule to be able to spend time with her family when she wished. It was all rapidly working out the way she had dreamed.

At this very point, however, she was struck for the first time in many years by an acute attack of back pain which left her barely able to return to my office for the third and fourth sessions.

Back pain is an indication of strong muscular tension caused by pronounced emotional stress. What had happened in those few days to create enough nervous tension to trigger a crisis so acute that she was hardly able to walk? Indeed, the pain was so intense that she was almost immobilized.

For more than sixty years Mrs. T.I. had cultivated attitudes of denial, omission, and distortion of her life, curtailing her activities and her progress, in a clear expression of extreme envy.

Certainly society also had considerable influence in that it helped to steer her away from personal realization, inasmuch as the social system itself is also founded on envy. The philosophy that governs human society is one in which no one wishes to make anyone else's progress easier. Nevertheless, why, precisely when she was being encouraged to do something worthwhile and liberating, did this woman show such strong resistance?

The answer can be found in the projective mechanism that many women develop; that is, they project their own resistance to progress, all of their own envious inactivity, upon their husbands, their children or society. And since they fail to perceive this resistance, this envy, in themselves, their sabotage continues unchecked.

Having passed the age of sixty, with her children grown, approval from her husband, support from her analyst and her friends, her time totally her own — in short, ideal conditions under which to do what she claimed she wanted to do — her opposition to happiness showed clearly and so her psychopathological picture became clear to her.

Women are known to be the most envious creatures of all. I would say, however, that they are extremely "inconscientized"; that is, they avoid all consciousness whatsoever, to take such a self-destructive attitude.

The well-known mother-in-law figure serves as a typical example of what I am saying. She invades the 'love nest,' using all kinds of intrigue and disturbing maneuvers that nearly always enable her to achieve her goal: to spoil the atmosphere for many hours, or days, or years — sometimes even for a lifetime. And why do daughters allow this to happen? Because they, too, have the same philosophy, the same belief that suffering is a necessary part of life. Some even reach the point of asking themselves: *How could I be happy when mother has so many problems?* or *Why should I have the right to enjoy life if my family is in such a bad situation?*

A 38-year-old woman patient, P.C., told me that during her childhood she had questioned why she should be happy, enjoy her toys and new clothes, and eat well when there were so many people suffering from hunger and cold in the world. She had wanted to be a missionary and be sent to a very poor country where she could experience hunger and poverty. To her way of thinking, she would thus be doing God's will by partaking of the suffering of other human beings.

At first glance the thought is a noble one, especially for a little girl of ten. However, deep down inside, what motivated this ideal was in great part her inability to enjoy parties and trips because she thought her mother and sister were unhappy. She saw it as a kind of "treason" if she were to "unfeelingly" ignore their unhappiness and she herself be happy.

Today I think about how insane this attitude of the human being is — and the more neurotic the individual, the greater his opposition to happiness. Obviously, we aren't fully aware that we do this nor, especially, are we aware that the underlying cause of this phenomenon is universal envy.

We believe that happiness is what we most desire in life. And what we most desire is precisely what we reject the most! Yes, human beings — men and women — become neurotic and psychotic because they are simply incapable of making an effort to enjoy the happiness that the Creator offers them. In addition, the most insane members of society do everything to prevent them from having it.

I am hopeful that once humanity becomes aware of the true cause of the question, people will change their attitudes and begin to take advantage of all the truly good things they were meant to enjoy.

2

What I Don't See Doesn't Exist

The human being believes that what he doesn't see doesn't exist. And women are the strongest followers of this philosophy, believing as they do that if they are alienated, detached from their problems, then everything will be all right in their lives. The worst of it is that this is the very idea that *does* ruin a woman's life, for by denying consciousness of her problems, she, in fact, denies the only thing that can help her.

I believe that in the last few decades women have taken some decisive steps toward broadening their awareness. The feminist movements and their leaders actually achieved something highly positive in their attempt to open women's eyes to economic, social and family problems.

There have been many advances. Women began to take greater interest not only in the social and economic situation of their families and of themselves but also in the situation of their country and the leaders who regulate the laws. They began to vote to choose their president, governor, mayor; they entered the universities and began to practice professions and support themselves and very often even their families. They have achieved equality with men in many ways.

And yet something is missing in this advance: a more careful analysis of the errors and difficulties of women themselves. A great deal of injustice and abuse has been denounced, and with this, many women were able to emancipate themselves. But we have overlooked one thing: self-criticism, which is very important, if not essential.

We have critized the injustice and unfairness with which men treat us, yet we have said little about ourselves. We position ourselves as victims who have done nothing to contribute to the unsatisfactory situation in which we find ourselves. This is why the book *The Cinderella Complex* became a best-seller and caused such repercussions. It was the first to focus on the woman's problem: her wish to live out a fairytale which leads to alienation and dependence on her supposed prince charming.

Men are accustomed to being criticized for their faults. Studies and more studies have been carried out to analyze male psychopathology. And it has done the men a world of good; it has enabled them to correct themselves in many ways and at least show some degree of constant evolution.

That is what we women have lacked — someone to criticize us and point out our real problems; someone who will force us to deal with the real cause of our problems so that we can develop. We are, indeed, in dire need of someone who will show us all of the things we are unwilling to see. And my hope is that this book will be of help in filling this need.

Another source of help for us is that the power-wielders, enemies of women (and of men), have begun to be denounced by Norberto R. Keppe in his book, *Liberation of the People — The Pathology of Power*. Once we have become aware of these problems, there will be great advances in our liberation.

3

Modern-day Eves

At the beginning, the Devil tempted Eve directly because he knew she was more susceptible to his enticement. And in the same way that he tempted her, he continues to entice women's minds into adoring themselves (narcissism) and adoring the megalomania of men.

If a woman pays attention to her thoughts, she will discover that 99 percent concern herself: what she can do to become more attractive, admired and loved. Except for the hours spent at work, when they are forced to concentrate on something useful, women fantasize constantly with themselves as the central figure.

A lot of women will rebel against what I say, unwilling to admit the truth of it. But those who are more honest will accept this awareness and feel deeply ashamed of their ridiculous attitude. They will begin to see the enchantment there is in life and in other people; in music, art, culture and nature; and especially in God — who possesses absolute beauty and perfection. Indeed, they will become enamored of Him.

It is also certain that a lot of people will try to prevent this from happening, beginning with those who are in some manner in league with the woman's narcissistic way of being. The many men who are involved in a relationship that is based on a pact of megalomania and narcissism will attempt to deter any such change, as will the many women who, out of envy, do not want to see the happiness and progress of their rivals — to say nothing of economic power, which exists for the most part at the expense of female craziness.

On the other hand, there are many who will be pleased — those many who have loved and good intentions in their hearts. They will look with pleasure at women who are liberating themselves, free of such heavy burdens, free of the woes that self-adoration engenders. They will see them improve and begin to integrate themselves into life, enter into activities, achieve realization, and even become more beautiful because of the affection (love) that will naturally overflow.

A woman must be like a flower, perfuming and enhancing society with all of her love, dedication, intelligence and sensibility directed outwardly toward others. She must not close herself as though she were in a cocoon, her eyes only on herself, turning ugly and witless and becoming cold, useless, selfish and coarse.

4

Each of Us Lives the Life We Think Best for Ourselves

For the most part, even though we may not be clearly aware of it, each of us has chosen the life we have because we consider it the most advantageous.

If we women are in a difficult situation, estranged from socio-economic reality, excluded from the so-called male world of realization, it is because we feel deep inside that this is the best way for us to live. Our philosophy of life, our thoughts and ideas, may be correct to a certain extent. They may even be consistent with the mainstream thinking of society. Yet what we *feel* is very often the opposite of what we *think*.

The point I wish to make is that we women feel that it is better for us to be alienated, removed from any real awareness of social, political, economic and even family problems. We believe that by acting like the proverbial ostrich, we will suffer no harm and someone will always be there to take care of us. As a result of this evasion we become like the insane: unbalanced, alienated, ignorant of the reality we should be aware of in order to defend ourselves from the ill-intentioned and the sharp-eyed hawks of power.

If human society is in a chaotic state, at least 50 percent of the blame is ours, for we women make up 51 percent of the world's population. Since the quality of life of a people depends on the degree of consciousness that people possesses, it follows that the poor quality of life of all humanity is due in great part to the alienated state in which we females have chosen to remain.

Let me try to exemplify. In her sessions of analysis, C.V., a woman patient, commented often about Michael, a young boy

25

who lived in her house and who was spoiled by his parents, his aunts and uncles, and friends of the family. C.V. showed a deep involvement with the boy — a mixture of irritation and constant worry, which was unjustifiable, since she was not related to him or in any way responsible for him, nor did she look after him. What bothered her most was Michael's spoiled attitude, hanging on his mother's apron strings, trailing around after her or, in her absence, after any other adult who was willing to cater to his dependence.

I asked the patient whether she realized that she identified herself with the boy, whether she was aware of the fact that she herself was dependent and spoiled, that she attached herself to one person after another, forever alienating herself, unwilling to take care of her own life and face her shortcomings.

She admitted that she could see this, and that she did not like responsibility or serious work; that even though she lived in a city like New York, full of opportunities for cultural and professional enrichment, she chose to remain distant from it all, isolated within the confines of her castle of fantasies.

Obviously, the results of this type of behavior are neither ennobling nor pleasant. Suffering is inevitable. The question that haunted her was why, if she was aware that her direction in life was wrong and she knew what she should do to become productive, did she do just the opposite?

Women fail to realize that they may *think* the right way, yet *feel* the opposite. In other words, rationally the woman thinks that awareness, responsibility, work, human relations and new horizons are preferable. And yet down deep inside she feels that if she opens herself to life, if she launches herself into new ventures, meets new people and new ideas, she will suffer; that is, that she will encounter more problems and feel ill at ease.

The truth is that each of us lives the life we consider the best, the most comfortable, because we often fail to see how dreadful the consequences will be.

The patient, C.V., believed that despite everything, her dependent, alienated existence, full of restrictions, was better than the life she would have if she faced the problems "out there" (outside her castle, her home). Believing that she would suffer far more if she opened herself to the world, she failed to see that out there, and only there, would she begin to feel really well and happy.

Women Fail to Develop Because They Lack Interest in Progress

A patient once came to her individual session of analysis to analyze why she was unable to concentrate when she tried to read the newspaper or serious scientific books that she knew were necessary for her development.

She said that every night before going to bed she picked up one of Norberto R. Keppe's books on Analytical Trilogy, books that dealt with her problems, and began to read. After a few lines, she found that she couldn't go on.

When I asked her why she wasn't able to continue reading, her reply was that she began to feel sleepy or started to think about her husband, her children, what she was going to do the following day, and so on. She had come to the conclusion that she simply was not interested in reading. I then asked her what she associated reading with, and the session continued with the following exchange:

Patient: *I associate reading with culture.*

I: *And these ideas that come into your thoughts when you begin to read; with what do you associate them?*

Patient: *Escape.*

I: *What you're saying, then, is that you run away from culture because you aren't interested in it.*

Patient: *Oh! The other day I heard someone say that when a person isn't able to read it's because of envy, but I didn't understand that. For example, I don't think I'm envious of Dr. Keppe. I admire him very much.*

> **I:** *But a person only envies what he admires!*
>
> **Patient:** *Really? How can that be? Doesn't the person who is envious want to be like the one he envies? I know I can't be like Dr. Keppe. He's far more learned and more capable. He's been studying about all this since he was young.*
>
> **I:** *No, envy means that you wish the other person were less than yourself. And as you see that the contrary is true, it bothers you and you don't want to see it. If you wanted to be like Dr. Keppe, then you would do what he does.*
>
> **Patient:** *Oh, but I think Dr. Keppe is enlightened. That's it; now I've found the right word: he is enlightened; chosen by God.*
>
> **I:** *See how your explanation proves your envy: you say he is enlightened, one of the chosen ones, and that this is why he is so capable — not because he has dedicated himself since he was young and made a great effort to achieve all that he has — something which you never wanted to do or were ever interested in. So you think: "No, his life is easy; studying and writing is easy for him, but it's difficult for me. He's enlightened, I'm not." In this way you belittle his merit, which is the result of his dedication and will power, and you don't want to admit your own disinterest and laziness.*

I believe that the economic powers-that-be are partially responsible for the situation, for they have established a pact with women that nourishes the woman's laziness and alienation. In this way women are kept in a state of backwardness and underdevelopment, not 'threatened' in any sense, for men with power are also envious of women and like to see them remain in this primitive condition of intellectual, affective and cultural arrest. It makes the men feel superior and enables them to keep women entirely under their control, serving their particular interests.

Everyone ends up paying a very high price for thinking that the primitive person is more manageable, easier to control. Nothing could be further from the truth! Much to the contrary. The male pays dearly for his woman's stupidity and ignorance, for she eventually becomes his bitter enemy and puts children, family and friends against him. After a time, the so-called 'home' becomes a battlefield from which the husband tries to stay as far away as possible!

Men fool themselves by thinking that the alienated woman, the woman who is detached from the real world, will not cause them problems. In fact, very often what the man really wants is to keep the woman from bringing him any consciousness of his own shortcomings, for if she ventures out into the real world she will have her eyes opened to many things that would otherwise pass unnoticed.

The man imagines, unknowlingly, that his adorable girlfriend, who treats him like a god prior to the marriage, careful not to point out any defect in him, will go on being that way as long as she remains isolated within the home.

What a tragic mistake! That same sweet, angelic girl, after seeing to it that her man is safely tied to her by means of a signed agreement with God (complete with witnesses to guarantee that he does not go back on his word!), soon begins to see him as the demon of the house. She blames him for all of the problems that arise — everything from her personal insatisfactions to the fact that the maid has given notice or the children are doing poorly in school.

I consider it fundamentally important that not only women but men as well become conscious of all of these problems that have been kept hidden, so that not only will women be forced to behave more humanely, with increased awareness and genuine affection, but also so that there can be happy marriages, with the woman and the man, side by side, no longer enemies to each other.

6

The Underdevelopment of Women

It was with a feeling of sadness upon looking through *Bartlett's Familiar Quotations*, that compendium of mankind's most meaningful utterances, that I observed that the overwhelming majority of the quotations were by men (92.77 percent), and only 7.23 percent by women.

Women might argue that this is but one more proof of male domination of the cultural world and men's sabotage of the fragile sex, their unwillingness to consider the things women say and do worthy of note. A lot of us might even claim that most of the authors of the selected quotations are males because the editors of the book are men.

But a closer look shows that the question is not this alone. In fact, of the few women cited, most of them speak mainly *about* women and *to* women. Whereas most of the men speak of social, philosophical, political and universal matters, topics that are of benefit to all people — men, women, children, the aged, the young — the women cited repeatedly contest, plead their cause, or speak out on subjects that are of interest only to women. This reflects the alienated attitude of the members of the so-called weaker sex who, in addition to being querulous much of the time, are interested mainly in themselves.

It is not difficult, then, to understand why so few women are deemed quotable in *Bartlett's* compendium and others. It reflects women's cultural marginalization, caused not only by the fact that the men in the "system" willfully exclude them, but also because the subjects women dwell on are of little interest and little use not only in the general social milieu but also to women themselves.

31

Indeed, I would far rather read quotations by someone such as Aristotle, Kant, Plato or Lincoln than by one of the feminists. For example, Anita Loos (1893-1981) made this "contribution" to female culture:

> *Kissing your hand may make you feel very very good,*
> *but a diamond and sapphire bracelet lasts forever.*

Her statement indicates clearly that her greatest concern in life was to acquire things that nourished her feeling of power.

There is nothing wrong in a woman's liking jewelry. The problem begins when she makes the acquisition of it one of the principle goals in her life, as many women do. I have had patients who spent twenty or thirty years of their lives waiting for the day when they would receive a diamond ring or a string of pearls.

We women are trained *not* to think, *not* to use our intelligence and our capabilities. It is in the interests of the power systems that the female be an obedient servant to the system, questioning nothing. And we are expected to serve power in various ways:

1. With dedicated, high quality work for low salaries;
2. Through the consumer system, by spending our money on things that make those who possess the power of money even richer;
3. By serving as an "accessory" in the life of powerful men, catering to their sexual or personal wishes in some way.

The worst part of all this is the fact that society has undergone a type of brainwashing that is designed to keep women alienated.

For example, in research carried out at the University of Southern California, a survey was made of 1,250 women graduates of Hunter College High School in New York between 1911 and 1983. (The minimum IQ for admittance to the school is 130.) The findings showed that:

> *The overwhelming majority of the women are home-*
> *makers or work at female-dominated low-paying jobs*
> *such as teaching. 'Given the extraordinary ability of*
> *these girls, there were remarkably few doing high-level*
> *policymaking anywhere,' said Betty Walker, U.S.C.*

education professor and a Hunter High alumna herself.
About ninety-eight percent of the alumnae were "ter-ribly critical" of the counseling they got at school. Many said they had left with no real understanding of their career options. The parents' expectations also con-tributed to their daughters' inexpressive future, the experts said. (USA Today, February 25, 1986).

Indeed, women have achieved less in our civilization, not because they are any less capable or any less intelligent than men, but because they concentrate their efforts in those areas that interest them. And since their interests are focused mainly on the world of fantasy, the world of romance — a type of alienation that caters to the interests of the economic powers-that-be — it follows that they strive to develop their skills in this area, working to perfect themselves in the art of male conquest, in fashion, even in how to become more superficial.

This all appears to me to be a diabolic game aimed at neutralizing the female, who, were she to focus her efforts on more realistic activities (economy, society, science, etc.), would be highly successful.

A patient of mine complained that she found it very difficult to concentrate on her work because she was lost in thoughts of paranoid jealousy of her husband. Her productivity and creativity were deeply effected. By concentrating 90 percent of her range of interest on her marital relationship — *Does he really love me?* — all of the extraordinary potential of her life went ignored.

Women usually try to attach themselves to a man, an institution, a group or some such entity, for the female is not accustomed to thinking for herself. To the contrary, she follows unquestioningly whatever her doctor, her priest or minister, or her boss tells her, right or wrong.

We women haven't learned to face life independently. We shy away from making major decisions because they mean having to take responsibility for making mistakes. Habituated as we are to following the ideas of others, we have in fact lost contact with our inner consciousness. And we have forfeited a great deal by doing this, for we follow all kinds of erroneous examples without question. When the doctor prescribes tranquilizers or strong antibiotics for our children, we follow his advice blindly. If he recommends surgery, we undergo it without questioning the possible intentions or incompetence of the doctor.

By using our intuition and common sense, we could avoid many problems for ourselves and our children. Apparently the female sex has relinquished direct contact with truth and the Creator in order to establish it through the minds of others. This appears to be one of the major causes of our present-day incapacity.

7

The Desire to Dominate Obstructs Our Progress

The young lady, M.L., a 23-year-old architect, worked as an interior decorator in the city of São Paulo, Brazil. Treated very well by the clients, who often invited her for lunch, dinner or outings, M.L. felt admired and respected in her social nucleus, even though her clients were not very important socially.

Then she received an invitation to live and work in New York. This meant that she would have to start over again there to build up a clientele, make a name for herself, and so on. Yet in spite of the fact that she liked the United States and knew this move would afford her an opportunity to develop professionally, she strongly opposed this step forward. She was deeply afraid of the idea, in spite of the fact that there were no concrete reasons for her fear. Besides having relatives in the New York area, she would be able to count on support from a large group of friends there.

In her sessions of analysis she associated life in New York with development and progress. Why, then, such fear? Because deep inside she realized that she would have to give up the business she had established in Brazil, and in New York she would be unknown in her field and, at least in the beginning, be seen as just one more human being among the many starting out.

Practically every human being, in his innermost self, harbors the desire to be important, to be great, to be ''on top,'' dominating the situation. This is seen to be true in all sorts of different situations — from millionaire Paul Getty, who felt he dominated in his particular area of life, to the way the foreman on a plantation in the hinterlands of Brazil feels among his co-workers.

The man generally seeks domination in social or professional areas. He wants to feel that in some way in his life he is considered ''the best,'' the most important — either by his subordinates or his pupils, by his wife and children or his girlfriend, or even, in the last instance, by his mother.

We women are no different in our desire to be important. However, we seek this mainly in the area of affect, within the family or with friends, boyfriends and such. There is a Brazilian saying that goes: *A woman will accept everything about the man she loves except another woman.* Children are not much of a problem in this respect (although many women are jealous of having to share the husband's love with the children), nor are alcohol, gambling or work. These are merely 'potential competitors' in the game of domination. Only another of our kind (another woman) can make us entirely dispensable in a man's life. This the woman does not accept.

And this is why our paranoia is focused mainly in this direction, for this is where we feel a threat exists to our affective domination of the man. From it come many of our fears: the threat of losing our security and having to regain — and *deserve* — the acceptance of others.

The feeling of security in a stratified and apparently stable situation keeps us from seeing clearly what we do. We stop 'checking on' ourselves, we stop comparing ourselves to others to see where we are failing, in what way we need to develop ourselves, in what area we must make a greater effort to improve.

I have treated a number of women in psychotherapy who used a legal document (the marriage contract) to maintain their artificial position of security and power over the members of their families. All of these women had reached a level of such blindness and alienation that they had become inhuman ''monsters,'' both physically and psychologically.

It is one thing to be considered the best mother in the world by my children, the best daughter in the world by my parents, and even, maybe, the best wife in the world by my husband, who is resigned to my defects. It is another thing altogether, however, to be a top professional in a situation where everyone has a chance to develop at the same time, in the competition for better jobs

or schools that are increasingly difficult to get into. In such circumstances we are constantly being checked on and compared,
with a cold eye and clear objective, to a score of other capable
individuals — and this invariably makes us feel so insecure that
we lose our ''domination'' of the situation.

I have seen many women who were reluctant to visit the place
where their husbands worked for fear of having their eyes opened,
fear of seeing too much. Perhaps all day long the husband has
women around him who are more attractive and more intelligent
than they, a situation that would make them feel deeply anxious,
realizing just how tenuous their position is as ''proprietress'' of
their man.

8

The Psychological Life of the Young Girl Is Basically the Same as that of the Adult Woman

Mrs. C.V. was worried because she could not concentrate when she was reading, and when she was studying she was unable to synthesize the materal because she failed to grasp the essential points. Encouraged by her husband and by analysis itself, she decided to go back to college, which she had left some years before.

At first she found it extremely hard to keep up with her classmates. She joined some study groups but avoided participating in their activities to any extent. She was a member of these groups in name only, for the other girls took it upon themselves to help her, writing the summaries, outlines, critiques and conclusions for her. When the study was finished, out of friendship they included her name on the list of collaborators. At exam time she was able to pass by cheating, either by smuggling a paper with the answers on it into the classroom under her skirt or by getting the answers from other students.

This whole situation left her extremely depressed, and she came to analysis complaining of her inability to study or work. I alerted her to the fact that if she had failed to develop her capacity for work and study it was because she must have other interests to which she dedicated her thoughts and energies.

Indeed, no one is "incapable"; we simply develop ourselves in different directions. Some head in the direction of reality, toward culture and love; others choose the path of deceit, dishonesty and fantasy, and develop the technique of lying to a fine art.

With great surprise, Mrs. C.V. answered:

C.V.   *But ever since I was a little girl, Dr. Cláudia, ever since I was in kindergarten, I've had these same difficulties!*

I   *Try to remember what your interests were at that time.*

C.V.   *Oh, that was such a long time ago...*

I   *Then try to discover what your thoughts are about today, what interests you, what you think about most of the time. That way you can tell in a general sense what you used to think about back then.*

C.V.   *Well... actually I just think about sexual fantasies. I think about how happy I would be if I could find a partner who loves me, someone with whom I could have a good sexual relationship. Scenes often come into my mind in which I'm kissing and hugging and exchanging caresses with a man. I'm constantly thinking about sex. (Pause)*
And that's not all! I just remembered that when I was little, there were a lot of boys around where I lived and went to school, and I was always off in a room somewhere with one of them, and we were touching each other sexually. While the other children were studying or out playing, I was always off somewhere else with the boys, "playing a-round." Yes... I guess what I did then is just what I do today. I'm that same little girl, off away from the others, always looking for a man who will satisfy me sexually, pay attention to me, be nice to me, caress me, praise me...

Note that all her life Mrs. C.V. was basically the same person: narcissistic, egoistic in her search for personal pleasures, interested solely in herself — an attitude which eventually made her incapable of participating either in social or professional activities.

Many women put the entire blame on society for their lack of independence, for the fact that they are not engaged in any social or professional activity. They are never willing to see that they themselves have no interest whatsoever in taking a more objective attitude focused on external reality. Rarely do they admit that their sole concerns have always been subjective: fantasies, megalomania, personal interests.

Another patient likewise commented that she had never been able to make choices or come to decisions. She said that she did not know what she ought to study or what profession she should follow. She thought she lacked some inner capacity to make decisions; that she 'lacked assurance.'

When I asked her whether she actually lacked the capacity to make a choice or whether she was never really interested in those things to begin with, she readily admitted to the latter, explaining that she had never really had any interest in the things that she considered to be of interest to men. She explained that she had never had any greater ideal or any idea of achieving anything more important in her life than finding a rich, cultured boyfriend whom she would eventually marry so that he would take care of her and support her — not because she thought she could not do this herself, but out of pure self-indulgence. Her wish was not to serve but to be served.

She admitted that during her whole life she had considered superfluous things important and had looked down on things of real value; that she had thrown away all of the good opportunities in her life, blindly and destructively, ever since she could remember.

Having later had the opportunity to analyze this woman's daughter, I noted a marked similarity in their psychological make-up. This is primarily due to the fact that daughters follow their mother's orientation mostly, just as they adopt the philosophy of life of those in their immediate surroundings and of the larger society in which they live.

The woman who has the opportunity to become aware of these problems early in life is able to overcome them far more easily.

9

Female Seductiveness

"Love a man like a god and be adored by him above all things." If the Devil spoke to Eve, I believe those were his words.

That was the beginning of the seduction that has been repeated generation after generation, with the woman praising her man as though he were a god, nourishing his fantasies and megalomania. "You are the god in my life; for you I will do anything. Be the greatest and best of all men and shine in the universe — but in return you must adore me above everything else in life and make me your goddess. If you don't (she thinks in secret), I will make your life hell."

This is where the infernal process begins. The woman demands the impossible from her loved one. First, she expects him to adore her above all other things, which does not occur because in many cases the man is more interested in adoring himself. And if, in fact, he is a truly affectionate person, then he will adore God first and love her at most as a human being.

Second, the woman expects of the man that absolute perfection and support that comes only from God. When the man fails to live up to her expectations (as has happened millions of times), she begins to retaliate in ways that are not easily tolerated.

At the outset of my training as an analyst, Dr. Keppe alerted me to the fact that there is always a very strong element of envy in the conduct of prostitutes and highly sex-oriented individuals. Later, having analyzed more deeply the behavior of women who maintain sexual relationships with married men, it became clear to me that they lead this type of life, not out of affection or mere sexual interest, but out of envy of the other woman, who is capable of preserving the interest and love of a man, and also out of envy of the tie of affection that exists between the couple, a tie which this type of woman hopes to destroy by coming between them.

Conquest in such cases reflects an extremely aggressive attitude toward the female rival and also toward the man, although very often the envy is hidden or masked by the romance; that is, by the sexual attraction and the fantasies they build up around the whole situation.

In many cases this type of woman will do everything she can to get the man she sees as belonging to another woman, separating him from his wife (or fiancee, or girlfriend) and from the family. But as soon as they take up life together and her envy is satiated, she loses all interest in her partner and begins to treat him with open contempt.

Another very important fact to be taken into consideration is that the human being can only establish a true dialectic — that is, he can only have a correct point of reference by which to orient himself in life — through God, who is Supreme Perfection, Absolute Good, Total Happiness.

The human being, no matter how good a person he or she may be, does not possess those things that can satisfy another human being. No matter how hard we may try, we are limited and very, very far from being what God is.

I find it incredible that after almost two millennia we still have not learned the lesson: The only way we can be happy, enjoy physical and mental health, achieve profissional, personal and social success, is by loving Beauty, Goodness and Truth (God) above all things, and our fellow beings as ourselves.

10

Narcissism and Megalomania

Narcissism and megalomania are characteristic of women in all cultures although, of course, such attitudes wear different guises from one people to another.

The Latin woman, for example, appears submissive and feminine, whereas her American counterpart seems independent and self-sufficient. Yet both aspire to the same thing: to have their personalities, and very often their bodies, adored by a man, by another woman, or by multitudes of people (i.e., American movie actresses, the girls on the beaches in Brazil, etc.). Indeed, it is no coincidence that the consumer goods industry is supported almost entirely by female narcissism and megalomania.

The "princesses" want to meet their "prince charmings" and establish their own little "kingdom" in the home. This pact of megalomania (adoration of one's own body and personality and the body and personality of another human being) is used by couples, both hetero- and homosexual, to avoid venerating that which truly deserves veneration: God and his whole creation, which includes the personal love relationship.

Instead, the majority choose to *exclude* God, who created everything and everyone; they turn their backs on the only being who truly possesses all of the infinite qualities to be adored. Only a very extraordinary being could have created a universe with planets, stars and billions of living beings, thousands of species of animals and plants of the most varied shapes and hues, a world so wondrously diverse, filled with surprises at every glance and every step of the way, created one day in an outpouring of love — this world that men destroy every day.

A Being so formidable, so loving and good, arouses two simultaneous reactions. The first is enormous admiration, even astonishment. Indeed, I get a giddy feeling, literally, whenever I try to contemplate the myriad facets of the Creator. The second feeling is one of disappointment, because in comparison to him we are nothing but a tiny speck in space; we see that beside him we haven't the least chance to shine as "special," "the best," "the most beautiful or charming." Nevertheless, all mankind will be enthralled the moment the people are willing to turn around and look directly at him.

With God we don't have much choice. Either we revere him and participate in his work, thereby becoming a tiny reflection of him with all of the happiness that love can bring us; or we become ridiculous beings: part human, part demon, exploding with arrogance and stupidity.

If you are really honest, as I am trying to be, you will see clearly what I am talking about. You will admit to this intimate, foolish, yet powerful wish to 'shine' (albeit for only a few fleeting moments) as *the* star, *the* light of the universe (even though many women consider their universe to be within the four walls of their home or their office).

It is precisely this desire that destroys our happiness, alienates us from reality and keeps us from experiencing the loveliest and most sublime romance there is: the love between a human being and God. It is this love that enables us to love everything and everyone without exception, for all other kinds of love are a consequence of this primordial love.

When we really love a man, we also love his children and all that he does. The same is true in regard to God. If we succeed in putting aside our megalomania and narcissism, we can love him very deeply, and this love will bring us such happiness that all else that comes from him (all that is good comes from God) we will also accept willingly.

11

The Woman's Liberation Will Not Come About Through the Libido

The woman makes a cult of sex in her life. She believes that affective-sexual realization is what will bring her happiness.

Freud was one of those responsible for the fact that this twisted, inverted idea prevails in Western society today. Nevertheless, the belief existed prior to Freud. Indeed, the fact that his ideas were so readily accepted was precisely because they reaffirmed what was already in everyone's mind.

Women protest, start movements, and mobilize their ranks in an attempt to eradicate their reputation as sex objects. And yet it is they themselves who nourish this farce. Although they may not be a sex object for a multitude of men, they are for at least one man (or one woman, if they are homosexual), and in this respect men serve as the means to their personal realization.

Fantasies of achieving happiness through another person inhabit the thoughts of all members of the ''weaker'' sex; from the time they are little girls, this idea is fostered in them by their mothers. All women believe that happiness and unhappiness come to them through a man. They project upon the man the entire burden of responsibility for their problems and frustrations, for which they themselves alone are to blame.

When I made the decision to write this book, I knew that it would meet with strong opposition from the majority of women, and no less from those many men who enjoy economic power and who maintain a silent pact with women, a pact based on their interest in keeping women in this horrible state of social, professional, psychological and cultural inferiority.

The female has been carefully protected by a 'halo' of sanctity both in the home and in society. Long known as the weaker sex — defenseless, symbols of affection, faithfulness, purity and self-sacrifice, women have thus been spared from having to suffer any consciousness of their pathology which, in fact, is immensely serious. And this is what finally led to the woman's downfall. Alienated from her shortcomings, not forced to face any awareness of her errors, which have long gone uncorrected, she sank lower and lower as each day passed.

Now the "weaker" sex fiercely places all of the blame for its problems and unhappiness on the "stronger" sex. In addition, society en masse endorses this show of female paranoia, leading women to see themselves as victims and martyrs when in reality they are far from being such. Present-day social and economic structures have obvious motives (which I comment on in other chapters) to encourage female insanity.

As long as women fail to recognize the catastrophic nature of the totally megalomanic and alienated position into which they have put themselves — living out a tragic fantasy in which they themselves are the sole prisoners — they are doomed to remain in a submissive position in society, a result of their incapacity and lack of equilibrium.

Some of the more imprudent men are interested in preserving this pact in order to go on seeing themselves as the sane, capable, balanced ones. Keeping women in an extremely pathological (alienated) state serves to nourish male vanity because men see that women — having relinquished reality, work and consciousness in exchange for fantasies — are, in fact, incapable.

Many people recognize the fact that women are more prone to fantasy than men, which is the same as saying that women are crazier, more unbalanced than men. Why, then, does society choose to perpetrate this deplorable situation, fostering as it does the woman's fantasy world, divorced from reality? This has to be corrected; it must be put aright immediately, for the harm it causes to everyone is very great.

Women, open your eyes to this terrible pact of destruction and death!

We can progress and improve our situation, we can be respected and admired, only if we are worthy of this! If we resolve to work seriously with the consciousness of our pathology (our envy, megalomania, laziness, libidinousness, destructiveness, projection), we can accomplish on this earth that which we have accomplished very little of until now: dignified work that is emminently worthwhile. Indeed, so very few women have distinguished themselves in the history of civilization!

How many women artists, composers, philosophers, scientists and others have made any significant contribution to mankind that we can remember? They can be counted on our fingers. And these women were not enemies of men; nor were they dependent on men. They were women who took charge of their lives with all that life implies: talent, opportunities, difficulties and, above all else, responsibility.

We hear a lot of talk today about women who want to "take charge," run their own lives. But what do they really understand this to mean? Their idea of running their own lives is to be able to do anything they wish — to be allowed to give all of their fantasy, all of their desires, all of their pathology free rein, total expression. And not rarely they confuse freedom with sexual liberation. Many who in the past suffered a great deal of censorship and repression in regard to sex, imagined that if they could put their sexual fantasies into practice, then they would surely attain happiness and thus be taking charge of their lives.

It is here that inversion of values came into the picture, the woman thinking (often with considerable envy and rancor) that men were happier and more privileged because they could put into practice all of the sexual fantasies that dwell in women's minds.

Despite the fact that they loudly condemned male infidelity, women nevertheless imagined that men enjoyed all sorts of pleasures and happiness that was denied to them for social and cultural reasons. They believed that the woman who was forced to live a life of chastity and fidelity was much more unhappy for this reason. Yet now that most women have indeed gained the freedom they so strongly craved (openly or secretly), they are neither happier nor more competent.

12

Women and Sex

In the past, the woman was considered an immaculate creature, a demi-saint to whom no pleasure of the senses was permitted. Sensual women were looked upon as exceptions and summarily isolated from society. Seen as sinners, absolutely incompatible with family life, they formed a class of their own — the prostitutes — on the outskirts of the social structure. Only men who were thirsty for sexual pleasures sought contact with them.

Since the decade of the 50's, not only has a great deal of progress has been made in regard to sexual questions, but the terrible censorship that existed has diminished. The sexual life of the female began to be looked upon as a reality to be studied scientifically, and even more important, to be considered a right the woman has to personal satisfaction and realization.

Yet, since for every strong action there is an opposing action of equal intensity, women went to the opposite extreme. They began to attribute an inordinate amount of importance to sex, which in reality is merely one aspect of life, and a secondary one at that.

So many studies have been done, so much research has been carried out, so much has been written and said in regard to female sexual behavior that, instead of women becoming more at ease in their intimate lives, additional anxieties have been added.

In the past, women were inhibited about their sexual needs and tried to repress them, hiding them from their companions and from themselves. For the honest woman, the mother, the wife, any experimentation having to do with the sexual instinct was prohibited.

In the wake of so many published studies concerning type and number of orgasms (vaginal, clitorial, multiple, etc.), the various forms of and positions for sexual relations, frequency of intercourse, and sexual preferences, women found themselves much more confused than before. To a certain extent, they acquired problems they didn't have before.

The fact that women consider sexual life a topic for special study shows that the woman still harbors considerable anxiety in regard to sex. Indeed, only those things that are complex, problematic and important require such a great deal of investigation.

Many women now become anguished because they make an effort to follow an "ideal" pattern of sexual behavior and, by so doing, destroy all of the natural spontaneity an instinctive act should possess. As an analyst, I have seen dozens of women who come, deeply afflicted, with questions they ask themselves and which they voice with great difficulty because of their censorship. Whereas in the past they worried about the fact that they felt sexual needs, they now worry about whether their sex life is normal, or whether they are sufficiently active according to the canons of modern sexology.

The kind of queries I hear from my patients are these: *I wonder if I have the right kind of orgasm; Is my orgasm vaginal or clitoral? Should I excite myself or should he do this? Is it possible that I'm just not as excitable as other women? Why don't I have multiple orgasms? Am I frigid? Could it be that my husband doesn't know how to excite me? I wonder if some other man would excite me more? Should I talk to him more about our sex life?*

Many similar questions began to fill the minds of the 'emancipated' women who now censor themselves for not being as sexually responsive as they "should" be!

Do you readers see that the censorship that formerly existed is still present, but under a different guise? What couple can maintain a satisfying sexual relationship in the midst of so many worries and doubts about it?

Many psychologists, doctors and psychiatrists recommend that couples talk over their needs, their likes and dislikes, etc. However, these long conversations merely build up tension and anxiety about something that is instinctive and natural.

Every person knows what he or she likes. Mary prefers roast beef; Peter knows he likes shrimp en brochette; and John's preference is stew. Even so, this is not sufficient reason to elaborate studies to determine how and why they like such dishes. It is natural and instinctive, and each of them knows quite well how to enjoy what he or she likes. Why then must we create such an odyssey in regard to sex?

I have verified the fact that the less a couple discusses sex, the better, because these long conversations create more problems than solutions. How, for instance, can a person relax if the whole time he or she is worrying about being tense and making a conscious effort not to be?

Obviously, education regarding sexual physiology is necessary, as is knowledge of the digestive system, the respiratory system or any other. However, the minutely detailed study of sex seems to be more a form of perversion than of science.

The excessive censorship of the question indicates that the human being puts too high a value on sex. We attribute to it a degree of importance which is absolutely disproportionate. Sex is entirely dispensable if a person decides so, and it can also be highly enjoyable if that person meets a partner for whom he or she feels a great deal of affection. But it will never occupy a primary position in the life of a balanced human being, who is more concerned with questions of realization and affection.

The true causes of happiness or unhappiness reside in other factors, psycho-social factors, not sexual ones. Sex-related problems result from the wish to escape from that which is fundamental: psychosocial pathology.

Individuals whose affective lives are satisfying, people who are contributing something worthwhile to society, those who are part of a more just, human and honest social structure, are calm about the question of sex and it becomes a natural part of their lives.

This is what we see happening in the trilogical residences, where people find their basic affective-social needs satisfied and become sexually calmer. In addition, their relationships are both healthier and more satisfying.

13

Narcissism Leads to Sexual Frigidity

The woman who is enamored of her body, who nurtures fantasies about using it to provide intense pleasure for her partner, or who has a great many erotic dreams, eventually becomes sexually frigid. This occurs because she concentrates all of her attention on herself and is not even aware of the other person. In fact, she does not imagine that there might be something in her partner to appreciate, enjoy and love.

Many women complain that their husbands are not skillful enough at love-making to stimulate them sexually, "that somewhere there must be a man who would appreciate all that she has to offer, who would love her as she deserves to be loved; a man who would know how to take immeasurable pleasure from her intimate parts..."

It is these same women who go from man to man in search of their Romeo, always disappointed at the end of each relationship. Some even try to fulfill their fantasy by way of homosexual involvements. "If no man has known how to love me as I deserve to be loved, if men are not sensitive enough to satisfy me, then may be another woman will." And at this point they venture into a path of infernal suffering, often unable to return.

Patient A.S. frequently complained that her husband was a very primitive person, highly impetuous and materialistic. She claimed that all he wanted from her was her body; that he saw her, not as a human being, but as a sex object, and that this not only irritated her but left her disinterested in sex as well.

After some time in analysis, she perceived that she was projecting her own idea onto her husband; that in fact it was she herself who thought only about her body and her ability to attract men sexually. Furthermore, she admitted that sexual attraction was the ploy she had used to lure her husband into marriage, and that very soon after the wedding not only had she begun to deny him sex, but she also became extremely irritated whenever he tried to approach her.

This same patient also told me that ever since she was a child, her family had encouraged her vanity by telling her how beautiful she was, and that early in life she had learned to take advantage of this. After finishing high school, she decided it would be better to get married and be supported by a husband who was well-off socially and professionally than to go on to college and have to make an effort to develop.

It becomes obvious that, for the most part, women prefer to be admired for their bodies (sexually) and their physical beauty than gain recognition for some worthwhile work, the realization of something beneficial for the family and society.

For centuries and centuries society has encouraged narcissism, leading the female to make herself the queen of vanity. Would not this explain why sexual frigidity is far more frequent in women than in men?

A number of people warned me that many women would despise me after reading this book, and many men, as well — men who are part of the pact, men who encourage women to see themselves as the goddesses of society. Nevertheless, I see no way out for us women except to make ourselves aware of the real causes that have led us to become so dependent on men, and not rarely even inferior to them.

14

The Woman Always Hides Behind a Man

What everyone finds most disagreeable and dishonest in female behavior is women's refusal to take full responsibility for their difficulties and problems. They are forever hiding behind someone, usually a man, to avoid responsibility for their lives and their mistakes.

Not infrequently women justify their lack of success by placing the blame on the restrictions of society, poorly-structured laws, absence of help from men, lack of support or limitations imposed on them by the family, and so on and on. The problem thus remains serious and insoluble, at least until the time when women come to their senses and decide to take full charge of their lives.

Obviously, many of the obstacles women cite are, in fact, very real. But the question to be asked in this: What is to be done about our problems? How can we possibly hope to solve them if we are not willing to take responsibility for our lives, our decisions, our errors?!

The woman imagines that if she does not accept responsibility for her life and the things she does, then she is not, in fact, responsible. She sees it as an option, something she can choose to do or not. Yet the question is that whether she assumes such responsibility or not, the woman *is* responsible for her life, her successes and insuccesses. Likewise she is responsible for her unfortunate choices, for the way she involves herself with unbalanced, ill-intentioned individuals, and for the way she relates to social problems.

I will attempt to exemplify this with the case of patient I.L., thirtyish and married, with two small daughters.

I.L. constantly complained of being unhappy and of having no chance to develop in life because neither her husband nor society gave her any help. In fact, she was living in a trilogical residence where she received all possible support from all of her fellow residents in regard to both her work and the education of her children.

Her husband, although not a person of any special merit, did pay half of the family's expenses and when possible helped her to meet her personal commitments when she was unemployed. Actually he was neither affectionate nor ambitious; rather the opposite. He was irresponsible in many ways and disinterested in work. The help he provided his wife and children was not graciously given.

And it was precisely this that I.L. used as a pretext behind which to hide, often complaining of not receiving more help from her husband, even in those tasks that were directly linked to her own work and responsibility.

One day I asked her what she would do if she were widowed at that very moment. Her reply — "I'd just have to manage by myself," — revealed the dishonesty and malice underlying her behavior.

Why does a woman think she can use this kind of excuse to justify her lack of development, her laziness?! All women should live their lives as though they were alone and solely responsible, even though they may live with someone.

If we women receive help from others, it's all to the good; but our existence is *our own* responsibility. For some very pathological reason, many women think they can make servants of their husbands and others. And if these fail to do for them what they themselves should do, such women don't take a step in any direction. And they do the same with their parents and with society.

Indeed, if we are exploited by our bosses, then we must start our own businesses! If our parents and husbands hold us back and refuse to support us in our undertakings, we must find other ways to accomplish what we want to do.

Women are unwilling to recognize the fact that it is they themselves who deny help to themselves, that it is they who shirk work and responsibility — precisely the things that can provide them with everything they desire: money, comfort, peace of mind, friends and freedom.

15

The Quest for Romance and Self-destruction

Have you noticed that when a couple begins to get more serious about each other they also begin to draw away from their friends and family, from their studies and other personal interests?

The man may stop practicing sports and give up the courses he once liked to take, stop seeing his college buddies or the group at the office. Not rarely he becomes sad, begins to drink more, spends more time watching TV, sleeps more, develops a paunch, worries more about money, and so on.

The woman also begins to see her friends less and less frequently and often stops working, gives up her studies or stashes her diploma away in a drawer. Alienated from the social, cultural and economic aspects of life, she begins to put on weight, loses her beauty and becomes dull-minded. Rarely does she recognize or admit any of this, until sooner or later the arguments between the couple begin.

The traditional structure of marriage and other affectionate relationships appears to be directly opposed to true human nature and genuine affective life.

I have observed that in almost all cases, when a person begins a romantic involvement, he or she automatically withdraws from all other areas of life. Both begin to evidence marked deterioration in regard to their friendships, culture, profession, spirituality and such. The person who is ''head over heels in love'' gives up practically everything else in life in an attempt to get the most enjoyment possible out of this tiny segment of his or her existence. By magnifying the importance of the romance, it becomes ''everything'' in life, totally out of proportion.

Nevertheless, we see that this is true of women far more often than it is of men. The woman destroys with greater facility all of her skills and talents, her career and her friendships, her spirituality — in short, the extraordinary gamut of experiences and options that life offers her — in exchange for romance.

No matter how good a relationship may be, it is impossible for a woman to cull all of the satisfaction life can afford from just this one small portion of it, this one facet of behavior. Obviously, the male-female relationship is an important aspect in our lives. But neither is it the *whole,* nor is it even the most important part.

When a woman abandons the other areas of interest in her life or relegates them to a secondary position, placing all of her expectations on a romantic relationship, she is committing a type of suicide — the most insane thing anyone can do. Indeed, it is no wonder that the results are always so disastrous.

This attitude, which in fact is highly pathological, is no more, no less than the woman's wish to destroy everything good in herself, together with all of the good things life has to offer her.

Such behavior is comparable to that of Eve, who, when tempted by the devil, forsook Paradise in exchange for the illusion of becoming a goddess. Isn't this the same pattern of behavior the woman is still following today? She turns away from the Paradise that lies before her — the thousands of options that would enable her to develop and have a fulfilling life — to gaze only at her 'god' in their little world apart.

What women do with their lives is a veritable crime — a form of alienation that has disastrous consequences for all concerned. Yet rarely do men do the same. Only the most unbalanced man ever abandons a career for romance — and isn't this exactly what women complain of: the fact that in spite of everything, men maintain a strong link with the real world, with humanity as a whole, and attribute less importance to an affective relationship than women do? Indeed, this is precisely what keeps men more balanced.

Really, it's a pity that women so often blame the man for the fact that the fantasy does not work out satisfactorily, for this merely serves to make the relationship more difficult by making it tense and even impracticable.

Each facet of life must be given its proper place, its due importance. How can we expect from a romantic relationship the satisfaction that we refuse to take from life itself? The fact is that each of us is but a grain of sand in constant evolution in comparison to the grandness of life, yet we want to be literally everything to our partner. Isn't this where the root of our inversion, our inverted sense of values, lies?

A lot of you will argue that men *like* to be treated like gods, adored by their female companions. True, most men do. The idea fascinates them, yet they don't treat their beloved the same way in return.

Be that as it may, such behavior on the part of so many women is not justifiable. It is a pact, albeit unspoken, that serves no purpose but to foment dissatisfaction on the part of both the man and the woman and generate an unbearable situation. A couple can relate well to each other only when they are united by a common goal that is superior — an ideal, a humanitarian undertaking, which gives their life together a higher objective than the mere union of the two.

In the words of Margaret Anderson (1893-1973), American publisher, ''In real love you want the other person's good. In romantic love you want the other person.''

16

Female Inversion: the Woman Sees the Truly Affectionate Man as a Cold Person, the Cold Man as an Affectionate Person

Many times I have asked myself why women in general prefer the type of man who is aggressive and ill intentioned (the most unbalanced, the sickest). More than a few women have come with stories of disastrous affairs, past loves which nevertheless began as great romances, and there have been many others who left their husbands and children for that "great love," which was soon to end painfully.

Can it be that the woman has dulled her ability to perceive things correctly? Is she unable to distinguish the worse man from the better? On how many occasions have you yourselves watched, astonished, as a situation evolved in which a woman of merit destroyed everything she had by getting involved with an aggressive, dishonest, self-seeking individual?

Only after I had analyzed many women who were facing this problem was I able to understand what occurs in such cases. The truly affectionate man is always dedicated to his work, conscious of his responsibilities. He is serious, faithful, and interested in doing well what ever he does. As a result, he has no time to give a lot of attention to women and he treats them naturally, like any other human being. In short, such men see no reason to pamper or coddle women.

In contrast, the man of bad intention is always ready to praise women. In fact, he spends a good part of his time thinking up ways to please women in order to attract them and hold them in his power. Such men scrutinize women's hearts and souls to discover what they like to hear and what pleases them most. Obviously, these men have little or no time to take care of the necessary things such as work, family, their fellow man, or the development of science or social welfare. Cold, calculating megalomaniacs, they are experts at creating a mask of affection.

The gallant, the present-giver, does what most pleases the woman — he treats her like a goddess. Yet it is short-lived, for the moment his capricious libido turns toward a more attractive 'goddess,' he doesn't hesitate to discard the one who now causes him problems and makes him uncomfortable.

A Brazilian patient of mine who travelled to the United States once told me how disappointed she was with what she saw and experienced while she was there. She complained of the "arrogance" of the American men because they treated women in such a cold way. Accustomed to being courted and complimented by Latin men, who are in the habit of flirting with women as they walk down the street, my patient found the attitude of the American male, who has neither time nor inclination to pay undue attention to women since his interest is focused primarily on the area of economics, very strange.

This same patient had had a boyfriend in the past who was seriously unbalanced, with all the characteristics of extreme possessiveness and paranoid jealousy. What led her to fall in love with him were those very attitudes of the 'impassioned man' — attentive day and night, bringing her presents and flowers, and the rest. Because of inexperience and ignorance of psychopathology, she was not aware that this constant control and desire to be with the woman all the time was nothing but extremely neurotic dependence, indicative of an extremely sick personality.

As time passed the man's paranoia increased and his deliriums multiplied to such a degree that he finally attacked her physically and actually came close to killing her.

Some three years later, the same patient met a man who was more serious, a well-balanced person dedicated to an activity that was useful to society. After they were married, she complained more and more frequently that he failed to give her the same amount of attention as the first boyfriend. She believed that a man in love should act as her psychotic boyfriend had. In reality, the affectionate man, the psychologically healthy man, is tranquil in regard to the woman he loves. He has no neurotic need or dependence in relation to her.

It is obvious that the woman who wants to be treated fancifully, who wants to satiate her narcissism, is going to feel deeply frustrated by a man with greater equilibrium who has other interests in life, such as accomplishing something significant for humanity. Many women cannot stand to be treated in a more normal, more balanced manner, because it forces them to see and feel their problems, their insatisfactions, which in fact have other origins. Sooner or later these women break off the relationship and seek a new one with a neurotic man.

17

The Woman Who Acts Like a Neurotic Child

A great many women think they are the same as children; that is, they think they can do whatever they wish and that society is obligated to accept them and support them.

The blame for this lies mainly with those individuals who cater to this absurd idea, fearful of creating greater problems if they fail to provide support for the women. And yet it is just the opposite: if everyone treated women the same way, pressuring them to become more mature and take responsibility for their errors as men must do, then we would witness great improvement in society in general.

I attended a patient, for example, who was already a grandmother. She had had five children and was married to a kind, hardworking man. Ever since they were newly wed, she had suffered constant bouts of depression and was afraid to go out of the house. She had never held a job, and in the home had always been lazy, totally dependent on maids.

In the education of her children she had failed completely, having allowed them to do whatever they wished, totally without discipline, and having set them against the father. The result: five maladjusted, useless people. Jealous and envious, she spent much of her time spying on her husband, sniffing his shirts for a trace of perfume, examining his pockets and personal belongings.

She had spent her life in the offices of psychoanalysts, priests and doctors, with her rosary of lamentations, often attacking her husband, creating intrigue, blaming him for her problems and pointing him out as the 'culprit' in front of everyone. Yet it was he who had patience with her, he who put up with her, calmed her, and resolved her problems.

Of course he was very much to blame in all this for having fostered his wife's aggressiveness and wickedness the whole time, thus preventing her from feeling for herself the consequences of her crazy, irresponsible behavior. This also gave the children the idea that they could do whatever they wished — shirk work, be aggressive, treat others with contempt, live an alienated life — and there would always be someone to provide for them and put up with their craziness.

To this day, now grown into adults, they are financially dependent on their father. In addition, it was very difficult for my patient to make any progress in analysis because every interpretation I gave her, aimed at leading her to adopt a healthier attitude, was nullified by the husband, who continued to pamper her and believe in her duplicity. (She frequently complained of not feeling well or developed some illness as a way of manipulating the family and getting her way.)

Such behavior is reminiscent of the attitude adopted by the spoiled child who, because he is unable to tolerate any sort of frustration, creates uncomfortable situations and is a cause for consternation in the family.

We are aware of the fact that there is a social pact for the purpose of keeping women alienated from society — a pact that was instituted in the interests of power, especially economic power. Nevertheless, the consequences that result from this type of conduct are equally traumatic for the woman and for the members of her family. The only solution is for everyone involved to force the woman into adopting a healthier attitude, just as we must do with a spoiled child.

18

Paranoia Between the Sexes

Men and women have been the victims of wholly erroneous orientation, maliciously engendered by the people who retain power. With a diabolic philosophy which they forged, the social and economic powers-that-be incite paranoia between the sexes, widening the gap between them and weakening both in order to dominate them more readily. While men and women are busy fighting each other, they serve the millionnaires and the powerful institutions without question. (In the chapter entitled "Women and Power" I analyze in detail the woman's role in these power structures.)

Women are in the habit of analyzing their situation in terms of "a male-oriented society," "a society of male values," "male economics" and similar labels that indicate that they view the question of sex as the cause of their problems. At the same time they fail to see that the majority of men are equally enslaved by socio-economic power.

Inadvertently the men themselves compact with the social injustices perpetrated against women, manipulated as they are by malevolent intellects in service to the dominating groups. Fathers and husbands have all helped, and in many instances still do help, unwittingly, to incarcerate in their own homes the women who work without remuneration of any kind, thereby indirectly benefitting those who exploit society.

Only the employee who has his food cooked, his clothes washed and ironed, his house cleaned, his children cared for, all for nothing, can survive on the miserable salary his employers pay him. If he had to pay the cost of labor for all that, today's economic situation would be totally different. The men would have to demand an increase of at least 200 percent to maintain the whole infrastructure that enables them to remain away from home in the service of their employers.

Look what has happened to people in the so-called civilized countries: The women who wanted to preserve a certain position of dignity for themselves and their families have been obliged to work outside the home because their husbands salaries are not sufficient to compensate for the exploitation wreaked upon the people by the economic power that has control over consumer goods such as food, clothing, home appliances, transportation, energy, etc., etc.

To the contrary of what many think, women found themselves obliged to hold two jobs, one inside the home, the other outside, working from 12 to 19 hours a day just to make ends meet — and still having to take care of the house and the children.

The ones most harmed by this are indeed the husbands and the children, in addition to the woman, obviously. And the culprits are not men in general (those husbands and fathers who are also sacrificed); the culprits are those who wield economic power — they may be men, women or both — under a silent pact.

Glamour, the American magazine for women, published the results of its "1986 Women's Views Survey," based on 800 interviews with women from 18 to 65 engaged in all areas of endeavor. The findings showed that:

> *Nearly 7 out of 10 women working full or part time outside the home reported worrying more about personal finances this year than last.*

The same article goes on to say that:

> *According to the Bureau of Labor Statistics, pay to the nation's working women advanced only a penny over 1984, giving them 61 cents relative to the dollar that a man earns. And professional women — those most likely to view their occupation as a career rather than merely a job — earned 75 cents to the male's dollar, up from 71 cents a year before.*

This shows clearly that there is a vicious cycle fueled by economic exploitation: the lower the income, the less conscious the working woman, and vice versa. Rarely can a woman in the low income bracket arrange the economic means to acquire the training she would need to cease being a mere exploited worker and become a 'professional' who can demand fairer pay for her labor.

In addition, we see that many of the women who went out valiantly in the 70's to conquer "a place in the sun" within the economic structure, are now beginning to be disillusioned. According to the forementioned study, 83 percent feel that they have fewer opportunities than men to earn the higher salaries, and nearly three-quarters (73%) think their chances for advancement in their jobs are smaller than men's. Seventy-seven percent recognize that they have less opportunity in politics than men, and 86 percent feel that female access to a political position is blocked.

The question to be asked, then, is: Are women in fact discriminated against by society, or are men more readily accepted and better paid because they are really more capable than their female counterparts?

I would say that both hypotheses are correct. First, the female has been greatly alienated by the social system, structured as it is to serve only the interests of small groups that wield socio-economic power. She has been educated to remain outside the system.

Secondly, because men have been educated either to do slave-type service or to be slave drivers (executives and managers who oblige the slaves to produce as much as possible for the lowest possible remuneration so that their employers will have higher profits and they themselves a few extra crumbs in their own pockets), they have in fact become more valuable to the economic structure the way it is organized.

As long as there is no interest on the part of the powerful, society will not provide the means for the woman to emerge from her present situation, integrate herself, and acquire the capacity to take a more dignified and active role as citizen, professional, mother, wife and human being.

My greatest concern is that neither the women nor the men are aware of the fact that there is no great abyss that separates the sexes, no gender gap. Instead, there is a huge gap between the powerful and the people, an abyss that enables the power-wielders to manipulate, divide, create dissent in order to enslave the people without interference. It is they who fabricated and who further the paranoia between the sexes.

While men and women fight each other, the real culprits — the exploiters and perpetrators of intrigue — remain outside, safe from attack. That is why that tiny minority has taken control of everything: education, medicine, psychology, publishing, the media, science, politics, business, commerce, and all kinds of trusts.

The people are, in fact, in the hands of perverse individuals and subject to a constant process of brainwashing that keeps them totally unaware of this reality. Conformed to the situation, they believe it to be irreversible, never imagining that true life is not like this nor that a very different kind of life can be had as of now. For this to happen, people simply have to become fully aware of the problem.*

* For a broader understanding of this, see *Liberation of the People — the Pathology of Power* by Norberto R. Keppe (New York: Proton Publishing House, Ltd., 1986).

19

Paranoia Toward Affection

The human being, male or female, is markedly paranoid in regard to affection. People fight against those they care for the most.

God created man and woman to be of "one flesh," meaning by this that he made them for each other, to live in close harmony and in such unity that their bodies would be one, as would their hearts and thoughts.

Why, then, have they become the greatest of enemies?

Basically, most couples love each other intensely. What upsets their relationship is the incredible paranoia toward genuine love that manifests itself in both of them.

The woman projects upon the man she loves the image of a person who can cause her a great deal of suffering because the love she feels is so strong that it is beyond her control. She then attempts to defend herself in whatever way she can from the one she feels is imminently dangerous, or rather, from that which is indisputably stronger than she. She fails to recognize that this dangerous element is not her partner, not the man himself, but rather the feeling she has for him.

For example, I have known a number of women who made it a point to marry men with whom they were not in love. They were looking for a more "tranquil," more "balanced" type of love, without ups and downs, free of jealousy and suffering and such. Little did they suspect that they were condemning themselves to disastrous marriages; for the most important ingredient was missing: genuine love.

The same holds true for men, except that they project on the woman *their* idea of love: something inferior. Many men marry women they recognize as good mothers or good cooks, not the ones who awaken their passion. Indeed, men harbor the inverted notion that love is an inferior element in their lives. Factors such as social position, wealth, power and assertiveness, for example, have a great deal of value to men, whereas the love a man feels for a woman is seen by him as something shameful and inferior, a thing to be kept secret, hidden from society, from himself even. The result is that his idea of the woman he loves is the same as his idea of the feeling: that she is inferior, weak, to be looked down upon.

Nevertheless this is also directly related to the paranoia the man feels in regard to love. He is deeply afraid to feel that something is stronger and more powerful than he is, to feel that love is also supreme in his life. He then identifies love with the loved one and feels indignant about being submissive to a woman, who is so inferior to him. He believes that by loving too much, he will become weak, impotent, humiliated, devoid of his assertiveness — that he will be putting himself at the mercy of a woman (instead of at the mercy of the love he possesses in his innermost self), and this he finds terrible. What will his friends think of him?

Thus begins the cycle of paranoia in regard to love:

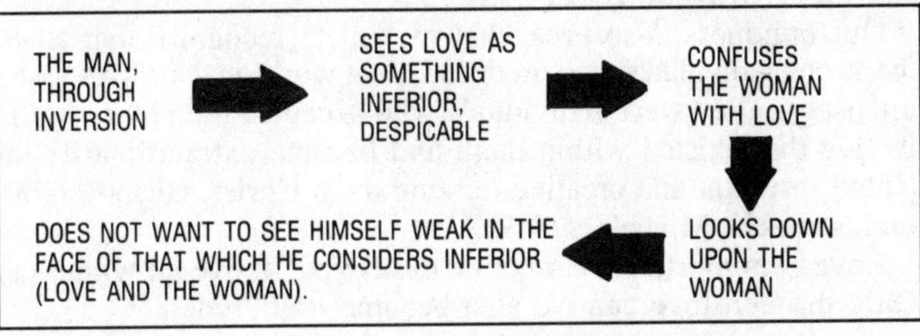

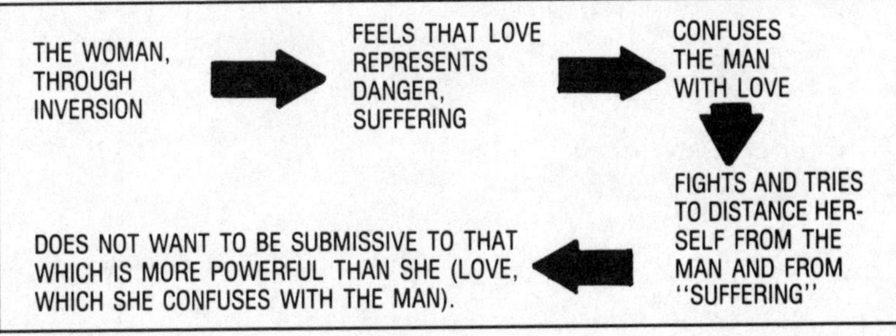

The story of Samson and Delilah, so often told to exemplify women's envy of men, also depicts male paranoia toward love — the belief men have that if they love, they will lose all of their power and become weak, the way Samson did when Delilah cut his hair.

We see here that the problem is one of inversion, an inversion of values, for it is precisely love, when accepted, that strengthens the life of the human being, man or woman.

Christ was clear when he declared that the greatest commandment of all was to love. Love toward God and all things, and toward others as oneself. We are not angels; we love with human love. And this love we feel for the opposite sex is no different from any other kind of love. Indeed, it is almost as genuine, as human and edifying, as the love we are capable of feeling for God.

When we love a person we feel that this sentiment is spontaneous — it comes into being without our wishing it or willing it. Springing as it does from our psychological nature, love cannot be an inferior thing or something to be feared. Yet we are willing to accept only that which *we* create and over which we have control, and this is why we reject love.

Our blindness is so great that we fail to recognize that all of the strong individuals who produced great works in their lives loved intensely. They were individuals who accepted the power of the feeling that existed within them and became extraordinarily talented, brilliant and creative (among them Christ, Ghandi, Confucius, Bach, Michelangelo).

Love is immortal. It cannot be destroyed, above all within us. Only through love can we also become immortal.

20

Marriage: The Woman's Profession

During my ten years as an analyst, in addition to my thirty-eight years of life, I have observed a number of things about female behavior that, unfortunately, are not the most comforting.

My observations have led me to conclude that the single most pathological attitude of women is their wish to make marriage (or a man) their profession, with the intention of gaining from it both financial and psychological sustenance.

Sometimes I ask myself where in the world women got the idea that men have the obligation to provide for them. Many of you would say that it is a question of education; that early in life the little girl is taught that one day she will be someone's wife, the mother of children and mistress of her home.

Rarely does one encounter a family who educates the daughter for life in the world at large. Girls are prepared only for a life within marriage, as though the so-called 'home' were the entire universe (when, in reality, in most cases it comes closer to being an arena than anything else).

Mothers begin early to teach their daughters to look for a husband who has all of the attributes that will enable the couple to lead a highly alienated life. The first prerequisite is that he be honest with the family but not necessarily with others. Second, he must be a hard worker so that the daughter will never have to go to work. Third, he must be a good father, which means he must be willing to look after the children whenever necessary and be responsible for the most difficult part of their education. Not only must he mete out punishment and pass judgment on report cards, he must also argue with the father of the boy next door when he comes over to complain of a broken window. And so on and on.

Fourth, he must be good-looking, as proof of the daughter's "worth" and also to provoke envy in other women. Fifth, he must act like a eunuch with other females, but be ready to satisfy the daughter whenever she so desires. Sixth, he must be of "good" family, especially one with a great deal of money, to ensure that the whims and caprices of her daughter will be attended to. And seventh, he must never ever, under any circumstances, go against the will of her "sweet little girl" or find any fault with her or her dear mother.

This is the way little girls begin to be taught to be like little goddesses. The next step is to set the girls against their father. With great envy, the woman induces the children to see their father as the one who is wrong, their enemy, the fault-finder, the 'crazy' one (if not the 'furious beast') that all of them must fear. The very person who supports the family, provides all of the necessities, pushes himself at great cost and effort to give the family all it needs, is very often looked upon as an adversary by his children. Furthermore, the father has neither the time nor the opportunity to rectify this image of himself since the mother is with the children most of the time, subtly, slyly scheming and sabotaging the father's character.

It doesn't take long to undermine the authority the father needs to educate his children. Because of her excessive envy, the woman works at destroying both: the man's image within the family, and the children's education.

With her contriving, in most instances it is the mother who is responsible for the fact that sons grow up to be useless individuals, criminals, mentally ill, or homosexuals, for by sabotaging the father's image, the mother prevents the children from seeing anything favorable in the example set by the hard-working father.

21

Marriages Fail Because They Are Pacts of Narcissism and Megalomania

Marriage is a pact of death because the man and the woman unite so that she can worship the power (megalomania) of her man and he can admire the body (narcissism) of his woman. Behind both attitudes lies self-worship, realized by each one through the other. This is why an overwhelming majority of marriages fail.

In most cases the woman demands absolute adoration from her husband and children — that is, when she is willing to share her husband's attention with children, for some women reject pregnancy without realizing it, becoming sterile in order to remain the center of attention.

On the other hand, many men want their wives to be beautiful, dependent and ignorant. It makes them feel important, indispensable — and the idea pleases them. They believe, ingenuously, that this type of woman will stay under their control.

Yet all of this costs both of them dearly! The truth of the matter is that the man becomes obliged to live with a useless, primitive, materialistic woman who is incapable of conversing about things that interest him because she knows nothing about anything except what concerns their little domestic kingdom. On our side, we women condemn ourselves to an unfulfilling life; we become alienated and unbalanced dealing only with children, animals, pots and pans, and shopping. This is why so many affective relationships end disastrously.

A woman once came to me to seek help because she was going through a terrible existential crisis. Sick and continually depressed, she found no joy in anything or anyone. Her husband was a typically megalomanic and materialistic man, and the couple's sole concern lay in achieving social recognition and accumulating material wealth.

Her time was spent planning parties or attending them, shopping for the latest fashions and make-up, being groomed at the beauty salon, or else travelling — all part of the pact of ostentation she had with her husband: the two of them in their little kingdom, trying to appear totally happy to others but behind closed doors suffering terrible anguish.

On the brink of separation, the couple lived in a climate of mutual hate. She blamed him for all of her suffering and could not stand to have sexual relations with him. This served to make the tension in the house even greater, and her despair eventually became so great that she fell seriously ill and had to be hospitalized.

After starting analysis, the couple came to realize that they had tried to create their own kingdom on earth, built around their private interests, and that this kept them from enjoying the kingdom that already exists; that is, real life.

When a couple lives for a common ideal and works for beauty, truth and goodness, then their relationship can be extremely harmonious and happy. This has been accomplished for the most part by couples who became aware of their theomania (wish to be all-powerful, God-like), and relinquished their fantasies of power to live for something real. The wishes of each became the wishes of both and their fighting thus ceased, because it had resulted from conflicting, contradictory wishes based on the woman's narcissistic attitudes and the man's megalomanic desire for power.

In general, marital conflict is always the same: the woman craves more attention, more money, more sex, more amusement; she nags the husband about his infidelity (real or imagined); and he, irritated by the situation at home, desperately seeks escape through fleeting affairs or in his work. Some men also fight to maintain their dominance within the home in the wish to make the wife and children forever dependent on him.

In most cases, however, the husband arrives home exhausted at the end of the day, ill-tempered as a result of his efforts in the struggle for power. After all this, he still has to face his wife's long list of laments, her endless complaints and the demands of the children.

Indeed, no one can stand such an infernal burden! Just keeping his own 'kingdom' together becomes the most difficult task of all. And all of this takes its toll in the many men who die an early death trying to shape reality to their imaginings.

When both wife and husband begin to strive for the ideals of peace, love and beauty above all else, they 'sacrifice' their personal vanities to achieve a common goal: happiness.

22

Why Do Men Lie to Women?

At social gatherings and in the workplace men tend to form all-male conversation groups, just as women usually do. It seems that male conversation runs on a different wavelength from that of females; the two sexes converse on different 'channels,' for not only are the topics they choose to discuss of little or no interest to the opposite sex, they are often incompatible as well.

Have you ever noticed that there are certain subjects that men usually discuss only among themselves, rarely in the presence of women? In fact, all of the decisions men consider most important, they prefer to talk over at a considerable distance from any female presence.

And they are right! Since most women are not well-balanced enough to deal with the truth, men find themselves forced to omit certain facts and even to lie outrightly to them.

Women get together in all-female groups, far from any man, in order to criticize men or complain about them — or else merely to chat about all sorts of female fantasies and futilities. Men get together far from female ears to discuss questions of primary importance to both sexes (and, of course, also to talk about women).

Very often women are kept from knowing anything about the more serious problems because, in addition to their not having the slightest idea of how to solve them, they become extremely upset and fearful, and this only makes it even more difficult to find a solution.

The one area in which men do allow women to take part in the discussion is when affective and family life is concerned, this being the female's sole interest. And even here, women create a great deal of confusion, pitting one person against another. Although considerable care is taken not to include women in any discussion of vitally important matters, when this is not possible, a great deal of effort is required to neutralize the woman's lack of balance.

I once overheard a man complain that women don't like the fact that men lie to them, but that they (the women) are never willing to hear the truth! If a man tells a woman the truth, he said, she gets so mad, her reaction is so unreasonable, so out of balance, and she argues so much, that he gives up trying and either goes about settling matters himself without telling her, or else he lies to her about it.

Why does a woman react this way? Because she becomes emotionally involved in all matters, and the result, in most cases, is that her reaction is unbalanced: she either argues and shouts, or she breaks into tears.

This type of female behavior merely serves to increase the distance between the man and the woman, he on one side, she on the other — understanding each other less and less as each day passes.

Men react in various ways toward women's intolerance, their unwillingness to face the truth and to recognize their mistakes and difficulties in general. The man may ask for a divorce; or he may give her enough money to keep her distracted, shopping and traveling. He may see to it that she stays at home, caring for the house and the children; or perhaps he finds a lover or some sort of vice that allows him to escape periodically. Again, he may simply decide to stay single forever.

When the children begin to grow up, they start to be conscious of the difficulty their father has had to face, because they, too, find they cannot tell their mother the truth without having her start an argument or become emotionally upset and make a scene.

It doesn't please me to see how unbalanced our sex has become. It will be very gratifying if those of you who are more honest and more willing to recognize the problem, change your attitude and help other women to do the same.

23

The Woman Imitates Her Mother's Affective Behavior

When the mother is loving and accepts her husband and men in general with ease, the daughter has a much better chance of also being open to affection in her life. When the opposite is true and the mother rejects the males of the household, then the daughter will have a great deal of difficulty in accepting her husband, boyfriend, companion, son or any other male, because girls imitate their mother's affectionate behavior.

A young woman patient, V.R., had a very serious problem in relating to males. Unable to approach them, she made friends only with other females, and even this was difficult for her. The fact that she had never had a boyfriend gave her a complex. At work she preferred a female supervisor, and when she decided to do psychoanalysis she looked only for female analysts.

The family in this case played an important role in the development of her neurotic behavior. Her mother, a schizophrenic, had been hospitalized a number of times. Her father, a depressive but kind individual, absorbed in spongelike fashion all of his envious wife's aggressiveness.

Early in life V.R. learned this insane behavior from her mother and she, too, began to attack her father in imitation of the mother's angry, envious conduct toward men.

In one particular session, V.R. brought up a question that was making her feel especially upset: the fact that she couldn't find a boyfriend. She claimed that none of the boys who interested her paid any attention to her. Upon deeper investigation, she admitted to having had a boyfriend for five years who finally left her for another girl whom he married a short while later.

Obviously, V.R. did not perceive that she alone was to blame for what had happened. However, I was able to guide her in analysis in such a way that I succeeded in leading her to see that the way she had behaved toward the boyfriend reflected such hatred and disdain, in imitation of her mother, that it had driven him from her life.

Recalling the past, she admitted to having attacked him openly for five years, with her mother's approval. The two women maintained a silent pact: the mother contemptuous toward the father; the daughter toward the boyfriend. Considering themselves superior to their companions, the two women created a climate of hostility that was unbearable for both men.

Obviously the boyfriend, no matter how masochistic he may have been, would have rebelled sooner or later against such open warfare. When he eventually found a more affectionate girl, he didn't hesitate to change one for the other. He was her first and last boyfriend.

When she admitted that she was filled with a feeling of hate when the boy left her, I went on to correct her, saying, ''No, it was when he left that you began to see just how much hatred you had always felt, the hatred that caused you to drive him away from you.''

The woman must recognize the fact that she imitates the negative behavior of her mother and other women in the family far more than she thinks. Many conjugal problems and others that seriously affect loving relationships could be avoided if the woman realized this in time. So often the wife treats the husband just like her mother treated her father — and she does it without realizing it. Indeed, she herself criticizes the disagreeable way her mother acts within the family.

Only through this heightened consciousness can a woman wake up to the grave errors she makes which ruin her life, errors she does not perceive.

24

Pacts

Speaking of pacts, it was Jean Jacques Rousseau who said, ''The man says what he knows, a woman says what will please,'' meaning, by this, that the woman doesn't worry about telling the truth, only about pleasing the person she is speaking to.

Because of this, women create all kinds of confusion and intrigue; for what pleases them is to hear gossip, the bad things that are said about others.

Even considering that there are women who are more kindly, rarely does one of them wish to displease anyone by speaking the truth, for very often the truth shows how insane human beings are.

Thus, from childhood on the woman protects herself and others from seeing problems and human evils for what they are, creating around herself a rose-tinted world of hypocrisy and alienation.

When I tell certain patients that they must break the silent pact they have made with men by being submissive, subservient and dependent in exchange for a life of social alienation and irresponsibility, I am not suggesting that they declare open battle on men, like victims in the hands of torturers. After all, if a pact exists, it means that both sides agree to it.

Very often women go from one extreme to the other. Either they connive with the negative attitudes of husbands, children and society at large, a position that is to a certain extent immoral, or else they choose a type of freedom which to them means freedom to be aggressive, freedom to do crazy things. They go from being 'devout' Pollyannas to a life of debauchery.

It is difficult for a woman to maintain a relationship without tacitly agreeing to things she knows are wrong. In fact, in less developed civilizations (Latin, Arab, Oriental), it is not at all uncommon for the wife to live for years — not working, not study-ing, not going out alone, suffering abuse in silence — in con-stant fear of displeasing her husband.

When these women realize the absurdity of their situation, many go to the opposite extreme. The home becomes a battlefield. They torment children and friends, refuse to subject themselves to any restriction of their wishes, and often they are the ones who de-mand divorce. They seem to want to experience all at once all of the fantasies they repressed before then.

Such an attitude lacks common sense. Obviously neither love, nor work, nor study can cause anyone harm, as long as the per-son does not lose his good sense and makes sure to examine his intentions.

The woman who tacitly agrees to suffer abuse at the hands of an aggressive, tyrannical male, in fact herself harbors a similar aggressive and destructive intent in relation to her own life. And because she is unaware of this, she projects all of her pathology upon the husband.

If she does not become aware of this, all of her subsequent deci-sions will follow the same destructive pattern. A separation or any other type of break at the social level will not solve anything as long as the root of the problem remains intact in her inmost self.

25

The Psychopathology of the Family

The woman repeats along various generations the neurotic behavior of the females in the family, the granddaughter copying the unhealthy behavior of her mother and grandmother, both of whom have imitated their mothers and grandmothers in turn.

R.M., married and mother of a nice little girl, moved to a foreign country when her husband was transferred there. At the outset, the couple were enthusiastic about having this opportunity to develop themselves. They also believed it would be an advantage for the little girl to live in a different culture, learn a new language, and so on.

During the first year, R.M. became irritated and dissatisfied with life in the new country and began to make things very unpleasant for her husband. Her repeated complaints about missing her mother and her family created a tense situation between the couple. When the year was up, she started insisting that they return to their country of origin, in spite of the fact that her husband did not intend to abandon his new business, which was showing considerable promise.

Without clearly realizing it, R.M. was creating an unbearable situation that could eventually lead to divorce. She was, in fact, repeating the behavior of her mother, a woman widowed while still very young, who had never remarried because she felt that being alone she could take better care of her children.

The truth is that neither mother nor daughter were able to accept life with a man. Alerted to this, R.M. began to concern herself more seriously with her hidden intentions, after which the relationship did, in fact, show considerable improvement.

Strangely enough, R.M.'s relationship with her mother was so close that she wept in desperation over having to be separated from her even though she was with her husband and her child. In fact, she showed a morbid dependence which was far more a reflection of a very strong psychopathic 'pact' between the two women than of a truly loving relationship.

The phenomenon is a common one: The woman marries but is unwilling to relinquish the position of daughter and become, instead, wife and mother. Such women preserve close ties with the family, especially with their mothers, and they try to impose this same type of life on their husbands and their children.

Obligatory luncheon with the wife's family on Sundays, parties with them at Christmas and on New Year's Eve, Mother's Day and Father's Day; the presence of the mother-in-law during all of the couple's major decision-making discussions — these are but a few examples of the sacrifices a woman forces upon the one who wants to share his life with *her*, not with her family. Because these mother-daughter pacts are nearly always founded on extremely sick, unbalanced motives, the female influence becomes extremely disagreeable in family relationships.

It is extraordinary how women succeed in creating such webs of power and emotional manipulation in the affective sphere of life. As I see it, it may at times be an even greater form of torture than the social and economic power wielded by men. Female power is exercised by means of emotional blackmail, touching upon the most intimate part of the human being: the feelings and the soul.

Because of this, the mothers of various girls who have come to me for analysis looked upon me as their worst enemy. As soon as the daughters began to make progress in analysis, they broke off the unhealthy pacts they had formed with their mothers, and insisted on a more mature, freer and more balanced relationship. Those mothers who were willing to see the problem and recognize it for what it was, developed along with the daughters. The others took the daughters from analysis (when the latter were dependent on the mother), or did everything they could to convince the girl of "the serious harm the treatment was causing to the family."

The girls who continued refused to be controlled and manipulated by their families. They wanted affection and friendship, not unhealthy pacts.

26

Behind Every Unbalanced Man There Is Always a Neurotic Mother

Dr A.C., a middle-aged dentist, came to analysis to try to resolve his problem of intense phobia. Unable to work or accomplish anything worthwhile without being overcome by a terrible feeling of anguish, he had become dependent on tranquilizers. Equally dependent on his wife, he went nowhere without her and had practically stopped working.

After one month of analysis, A.C. was no longer taking tranquilizers. A short while later he was able to make the 3-hour trip alone from his home to São Paulo. Having made considerable progress in the process of becoming independent, he was soon able to resume work at the office.

Even so, his persecutory anxiety in relation to work remained, albeit in latent form, seriously jeopardizing his efficiency. At this point in analysis, A.C. began to recognize the fact that his mother had been an extremely important and dominating figure in his life. He was the baby of the family, twelve years younger than his youngest brother, who died under traumatic circumstances while A.C. was still an infant. The mother, a strongly possessive, neurotic personality, began to be overly attentive and over-protective. By helping him with all of his homework and catering to all of his whims, she had led him to believe that life, reality, serious study and work were threatening and burdensome — that they represented a great sacrifice.

A.C. admitted that he had identified with his mother's way of thinking and had adopted the inverted idea — a feminine idea, to be sure — that work is wearisome and onerous. How could he, then, accept with good grace something that deep inside he believed to be distasteful and wearing? With this idea firmly implanted in him, and without his perceiving it, he harbored deep opposition to work. It was this that caused him to feel such anxiety, such anguish.

Man's essence is his capacity for creative realization. The human being is basically what he *does*, not what he *thinks*. Thus, if an individual blocks an action because he thinks of it as unwholesome, then he in fact stifles his very essence and he will invariably develop terrible anguish and phobias.

God created us to be like him in our behavior. He granted us the honor of participating in the universal creative process, completing it and perfecting it. The only way we can become really like him is by doing just that.

Readers please take note: Mothers who pamper their children, leading them to believe that work is a sacrifice, that it causes stress, or that they must protect themselves from the world and from "others" because those others are enemies, are, although they may not be clearly aware of it, working directly *against* their children.

In English we use the word *spoil* to express very accurately what mothers, out of unconscious envy, wish to do to their children and, in reality, what they *do* do to them.

In the United States, the number of homosexuals has increased fearfully over the past ten years. Some statistics show that as many as 50 percent of the single men in San Francisco and New York (the biggest homosexual centers) are homosexuals. And this estimate does not include the many married men who are bisexual.

The figure does, however, coincide with the increase in one-parent families headed by the mother. Indeed, studies show that 30 percent of American families are 'female-headed' today. This means that 30 percent of the male children in American families are denied a paternal model to which they can identify positively, so necessary during the period in which a boy's personality is maturing. Boys who live only with their mothers often acquire the notion that it is better to be feminine, because they have no male role model to follow and know nothing about a really mature man.

Yet the most troublesome aspect of this situation is the fact that, in most cases, the boy also acquires his mother's negative idea toward males. Not rarely the divorcee harbors, often without realizing it, an extremely negative concept of the man who is the father of her child. Consciously or unconsciously, she transmits this negative image to her sons. Later, this may lead to serious problems such as homosexuality, insomuch as the boy becomes horrified of being a man like the one who caused his mother, the most important affective figure in his life, such pain.

27

The Woman Raises Her Children to Be as Useless and Alienated as She Is

The woman who is not clearly aware of her negative, destructive attitudes (i.e., her psychopathology), the mother who cannot see her faults, causes her children incalculable harm.

A mother educates her offspring according to her own set of values, her own philosophy of life, her personal experience. She doesn't stop to consider that she herself may be strongly alienated or, indeed, that her ideas of what is good for the children may not, in fact, be the best. Much less does she realize that they were not the best for her either.

Since girls are nearly always raised to be alienated, set apart from the mainstream of life, expected only to study and wait for a husband, but never to truly experience the value of serious work like that done by people who support themselves, as mothers they hold to the belief that this is also the best kind of life for *their* children.

My patient, B.P., 29, is a good example. After finishing college, he decided to move to another country and begin life differently. It was the first time he had lived away from home, and the experience of having to support himself was unknown to him.

So great were the difficulties he had to overcome, and so greatly did he suffer before he began to adapt, that if he had not been undergoing psychoanalysis, he would surely have succumbed and given up the whole idea.

In view of the fact that now he was feeling it violently difficult to adapt to the world, B.P. confessed that he had never imagined what a difference his not having had any work experience during adolescence could make. Nothing of the sort had befallen his friends who started working at the age of 13 or 14 while they were going to school.

Feeling disillusioned, B.P. explained that his mother had not permitted him to work while he was in school. Her argument went something like this: ''Now is the time for you to apply yourself seriously to your studies, not to work. If you don't take them seriously now, you'll be sorry in the future. Now is the time to study. Later there'll be plenty of time to work.''

At the same time, B.P.'s father, a man of culture who also had considerable practical experience in life, did not disagree with his son's idea of working. He knew how important work experience is for a person, mainly to integrate the concepts learned in school. He was aware that top students rarely became good professionals, a fact which demonstrates how harmful intellectualization can be in the formation of a personality.

As a young boy, B.P. wanted to go to work as an office boy. His mother indignantly refused to allow it because she considered her son too good for that kind of job. She argued that in addition to not learning anything from such work, he would be subject to all sorts of humiliation and danger.

We see here that the mother, imagining herself in B.P's place, projected upon her son her own fear of work, which she considered humiliating and useless. Her ideal was to be 'powerful' in society, married to a man more ambitious than her husband. She would not permit her children to do those things she thought would jeopardize her and them.

The fact is that B.P.'s mother brought her children up the best way she could, considering her criteria of values. She herself was a useless person who had studied and worked for a short while and then married early, thereby transferring her dependence on her parents to her husband. Seeing nothing wrong in this conduct, she wanted her children to follow suit.

The person who doesn't begin working early in life rarely succeeds later on. Bound to experience enormous difficulties in accomplishing anything worthwhile, he will have to face terrible anguish, as we saw in the foregoing case, due to the situation created by the mother, with the acquiescence of society.

28

Gossip: The Woman's Crime

If it can be said that any defect is typically feminine, then intrigue is it. When a woman opens her mouth to speak to her husband, her children or her friends, ninety percent of what she says is made up of malicious remarks about other people.

When a woman speaks, we always have to ask ourselves whether what she is saying is the truth or simply what she wants us to believe.

The most destructive weapon the female possesses is her tongue, which she uses to manifest all of the malice, venom and envy she harbors in her heart. At times subtly, with a voice of velvet in a tone that implies that she merely wants to help, she uses the opportunity to pour forth her fury by gossiping about others. Indeed, she is able to turn everyone against the person she envies, and very often that person is her husband or her best friend.

Unfortunately, it must be recognized that the majority of women are envious of just about everything. Further, they are not even aware of the fact — which serves only to aggravate the situation.

At the office it is always the women who gossip. The same is true at home, within the family, at the club, among friends, at school and in college. In the women's restrooms at these places you will note, if you pay attention, that there is usually a little group of girls or women gossiping about someone. Speaking ill of others is definitely a female trait — so much so that, other than women, only a few male homosexuals, in imitation of their mothers, also have poisonous tongues and take pleasure in seeing the image of others destroyed.

The intent to separate couples and to separate men from their friends, women from theirs, or to put colleagues in a bad light with bosses or teachers, stems directly from women's envy, of which they are unaware. What better way to 'eliminate' a female rival in the battle for attention or importance than by spreading gossip about her? What better way to feel superior to others than by talking about their shortcomings?

It saddens me to have confirmed through my experience as a psychoanalyst that women are decidedly the greatest slanderers. It is women who contrive malicious gossip, who sully the reputation of friends and members of the family with pleasure — a pleasure that only demons could feel.

A single calumnious remark, a single word of gossip, can do far more harm than physical aggression. A woman's evil tongue is the most dangerous weapon of all. Indeed, a person can easily be cured of a blow, a knife wound, even a bullet wound sometimes, but malicious gossip, calumny, is never totally erased. An individual's entire life can be ruined by a woman's gossip.

In this particular, the woman is reminiscent of the devil — often referred to as ''the slanderer'' — who through all eternity tries to pit God against human beings and human beings against each other.

Both women and devils try to separate, to hurt, slander, and lie, to destroy reputations for the pleasure of seeing their envy satiated. They are, in fact, unable to hold it in check.

I do not refer only to women who are seriously disturbed; I am speaking of the common female, who, although she may try to disguise her evil tongue, inevitably adds a little venom to her words.

I hope that my readers are honest enough to recognize this problem, for, because of it, women have been responsible for causing incalculable harm behind the scenes in all civilizations. Like witches disguised as angels, women hide themselves behind men and prod them to hatred, revenge and aggression.

One of the greatest difficulties the psychoanalyst faces is to 'filter' what the patient says about other people, which is almost never impartial or objective. Most of the time what women say is said for a reason. In the wish to gain some selfish end, they offer the rendition that interests them. By adding personal opinions and judgments, the woman tries to steer the story in a certain direction so that the listener is influenced against the person of whom she is speaking.

An example of this is the statement made by patient M.F. concerning a colleague, to the effect that he was incorrigible. "He's the only one who doesn't help with the cleaning and straightening up of the residences," she said, pointing to the person's laziness and arrogance.

When I asked her why she said that and how she knew it was true, who had told her, she answered, "Nobody said anything. It's just my opinion because I've never seen him do any work."

Clearly M.F.'s intention was to create mistrust and dislike toward the person in question, for she was making an inference, expressing what her envy led her to believe. The simple fact that she had never seen him working around the house did not give her the right to conclude that he never did anything. In fact, couldn't he have been doing his part some other place out of her sight?

You yourselves can test this. Begin to pay attention to what women (and yourselves) say: question it even though the woman speaking may seem very sure of herself. You will discover an incredible world of lies, fantasies and slander that you never imagined existed!

29

Women and Aloneness

Nothing is more disagreeable than the company of the solitary woman. Indeed, she is alone not because she has been rejected for no reason at all, but because she creates such unpleasant situations that living with her becomes unbearable. These women are usually so aggressive that people are repulsed and prefer to stay away from them. Even though the solitary woman nearly always has a family or at least some relatives, they prefer to keep their distance, and this serves to reaffirm even more strongly the idea that she is a victim of society.

If we analyze the situation more closely, we find that such females are careless in their habits, irascible, highly arrogant and aggressive, and that they blame everyone else for their problems and their suffering. Nevertheless, what they are really complaining about is the fact that they are not being treated like goddesses. Because their families and society in general are looking out for their own interests, the woman's selfish, narcissistic feelings are frustrated.

Mrs. P.E., a middle-aged woman from Central America who had been living and working in New York for many years, came to analysis because of the bouts of anguish and deeply disturbing psychosomatic symptoms she was suffering: symptoms that included dizziness, visual difficulties, headaches and others. Her story was the following.

Middle-aged and divorced, she had two adult children, one married, one single. Always alone, suspicious of everyone, she had just suffered a great disillusion in her love life. Having met and fallen in love with a man where she worked, she nourished the fantasy that he was in love with her, too, and that soon they would live and work together.

A short time after the relationship became closer, he confessed to her that he was a homosexual. This revelation set off such a strong emotional reaction in P.C. that the resulting crisis led her to seek help through analysis. Medicated with tranquilizers, she was unable to continue working.

If we look at the question from her point of view, we see a woman alone, the victim of her former husband's meanness and ingratitude after she had dedicated half her life to him; a victim of the indifference of her children who abandoned her for their own selfish interests; and now, a victim of the inconsistency of her new love. Indeed, life had seemingly not been at all good to her.

But if we analyze the situation behind her story, we discover that P.E., although unaware of it, had always rejected love, intuitively forming close relationships with strongly pathological types of persons and passing up the healthier ones. In addition to this emotional (affective) inversion which led her to distrust and reject true friends and seek out adverse personalities, she followed a philosophy of life which she learned from her mother and her grandmother. In fact, it was a "philosophy of suffering," a belief that the worthy woman is the woman who suffers, while happiness and a good life are the lot of the frivolous, reserved for women of no account.

This led P.C. to adopt an attitude toward life that was so negative and oppressive that not even her children could stand her presence. In defense of their own well-being, they kept away from her. As this served to make her even more reproachful, the vicious cycle was set in motion, increasing her loneliness.

The demands of the solitary female are far greater than those of any ordinary person. Jealous and envious, she insists on being the center of attention and is incapable of sharing the affection of her loved one with anyone else. Unable to tolerate any contradiction, not even the slightest frustration, she must have her whims catered to.

As girlfriends, such women absorb the man entirely, isolating him from his friends, his work, his family. Even his thoughts are kept under surveillance.

As wives, they demand that the husband treat them as though they were the center of their lives, the principal object. If they could, they would keep the husband at home. But since this is not feasible (otherwise they would die of hunger, and besides, they want the money he makes), they keep track of the time he leaves home, when he returns, where he went, who he was thinking about, etc., etc., etc. When the husband is at home, she nags him constantly, making life so hellish that eventually he gives up and may literally disappear in order to keep her from ever finding him.

The result: The woman, in a fury, her narcissism frustrated, seeks out their friends (usually *his*), relatives and the family doctor or clergyman to complain to and lament "the great injustice and ingratitude toward one who was so dedicated and has reaped loneliness in return." It is not long before such women succeed in driving even these friends and relatives away.

In reality the phenomenon is rooted in the fact that the solitary woman always considers herself perfect! And it is truly a phenomenon, for if she were as she makes herself out to be, a lot of people would be avid for the chance to enjoy at least a little of her kindness and affection! Why isn't this the case then, she wonders.

Such women may fool even themselves, and they may have as allies a few people who don't live with them constantly and thus have not as yet been caught in their tentacles. But woe to the one she has chosen as her target, for life at the side of the "solitary" female is absolutely unbearable.

This type of problem can be solved only by organizing society differently so that women can live in communities that offer them a chance for real accomplishment, a place where they can channel their affection into worthwhile action for society and where their inner potential can be properly used.

It is almost impossible for a human being to be emotionally fulfilled in present-day society the way it is organized, for there is no way the individual can direct his affective energies freely and in a healthy way.

The human affective potential is enormous. When it cannot be utilized correctly through useful action that is keyed to genuine science, art and culture, it inevitably ends up being concentrated in a pathological manner in a very small number of relationships.

Part II

A Study of Sociopathology

1

The Influence of Theomania in Education

Society functions like a mold which shapes the boy to be the best and the most powerful in whatever he does and the girl to be the most beautiful, charming and seductive of creatures. Man's insanity has reached such a level that the entire structure of life revolves around theomania.

Because of this, anyone who wishes to adopt healthier behavior, whose conduct is keyed more closely to reality — anyone who desires to progress toward greater well-being and happiness for mankind, and who is thus more honest and genuine — is automatically rejected.

The more affectionate boy, for example, the one who is neither interested in having a 'harem' of girls around him nor cares about showing off with cars, motorcycles or drugs, is considered abnormal and is shunned by the other boys. Similarly, the girl with greater equilibrium, the one who is less vain, is not readily accepted by either girls or boys. It is always the craziest children and young people who are chosen by their peers as leaders.

Similarly, fathers take it upon themselves to guide their sons along the same path: the search for power, fame and wealth; while mothers teach their daughters to be self-conscious and egocentric, fostering their narcissistic attitudes and giving them a totally distorted view of life in which they are to be fulfilled by becoming someone's wife.

Pay attention to girls' conversations right from the time they are little. They seem to be in a constant state of envy of each other. First, two or three group together and talk behind the backs of the others girls. Then each girl changes over to a different group and talks about the ones in whom she confided in the first place.

101

In the attempt to prevent anyone from outshining her, each girl tries to show that the others have faults. Thus, early in life female competition and intrigue gain such momentum that I once heard someone say that a woman's worst enemy is another woman.

Apparently we females can never trust others of our sex. Since the time I was a child, I learned that my best friends were mostly men.

However, by far the most worrisome element is the pact of hypocrisy sustained by families with regard to their children. A child is a social being who should be educated and ''molded'' by society, and yet mothers are incapable of having anyone else correct their children without feeling offended and indignant.

How often, at a birthday party for example, does it happen that everyone feels uncomfortable seeing the ruinous mess that ''little Johnny'' is making in the home of the hostess under the proud, approving gaze of his mother? Or how often have neighbors looked with pity at the middle-aged couple who are totally unaware of the gossip and piquant comments going around the neighborhood about their adolescent daughter who is being passed from one boy to another?

Although other people perceive much more about the children than the parents do, they can do nothing to help without risking being considered meddlesome and losing a friendship of years because of a few words. The truth is that mothers protect their children with feline ferocity from all awareness of their errors and shortcomings, keeping them far from the world of reality, like demented nobility.

It would be so much easier if other people were allowed to help educate every child and adolescent! If mothers permitted this, it would be of inestimable help and a great relief. The mothers themselves would suffer far less wear and tear in their efforts to guide the children along a more realistic path — an impossible taks for a mother alone with adolescent children.

Daughters who are excessively pampered are never able to adjust to any sort of real life in which they have to face the problems that befall all human beings.

Indeed, such girls become grotesque creatures, deluded about themselves and about others. Can you remember having known women who seemed to live in a dream world as they grew older, remaining at the emotional level of a 9 or 10-year-old? Do you recall how careful everyone was not to destroy the dream castle these women lived in so as to avoid disillusioning them or perhaps triggering a severe emotional crisis?

It is truly shocking to see how false society at large is in regard to women, forever pretending that it believes in the fantasies the woman forges (with her mother's help) about herself and others.

Society Helps to Spoil Women

The education women receive prompts them to follow a narcissistic philosophy of life. From the moment of birth, girls are taught by their parents and society, and later by their husbands, to value their mask and cultivate their vanity.

The little girl is more than used to hearing comments such as: "See how cute she is!" — "What beautiful eyes!" — "What lovely hair!" — "What a sweet child!" — comments which lead her to believe that her primary value as a human being lies in her appearance, her body, her physical beauty, not in her good actions.

With boys it's different. From the beginning they are treated with greater firmness. The least sign of vanity is eradicated at the start with admonitions like: "What's this, Joey? You're not a girl. You mustn't act like that. That's only for girls!" And this is to their great advantage, for boys learn while still very young that their merit lies not in their physical beauty or mask but in their accomplishments, their ideas, their intelligence and capacity, and their kindness toward others.

From a tender age the girl's vanity and narcissism are encouraged, while the boy is taught to work. And any boy who acts a little different is promptly checked by being called a sissy or girlish, all of which helps to keep him from becoming alienated, from losing sight of the true purpose of life, as the girl does.

Instead, he learns to take an interest in life, in others, in reality, conscious of the fact that one day he will have to work to support himself and his family and do well in some particular area if he wants to be respected.

A lot of you may argue that men generally think of nothing but earning money. I agree, and I find it lamentable. Nevertheless, to earn money in a competitive society, a person has to develop some skill or capacity of sufficient interest to society to enable him to "sell" his product, his idea or his labor. Unless he is one of the few powerful millionnaires in the word, he cannot afford to be very crazy, very unbalanced, if he wants to earn a living.

The woman, on the other hand, doesn't have to worry about any of this. She is raised to believe that most probably her mate will support her. Or perhaps that she will be able to live on what she inherits from her father. In the absence of either of these options, she can still count on the fact that men will establish businesses, schools and other social structures that can provide her with a safe, well-paid job — in most instances without any responsibiiity whatsoever on her part of having to set up an enterprise and run it.

This being the case, her interest is focused on what clothes she should wear, what makeup to use, what hair style is best, what tone of voice will enhance "her type" most effectively. Competition among females takes place mainly on this level. Women try to attract attention not by what they have accomplished socially for the good of others, but by the way they look.

Everything the woman sees she immediately relates to herself with the thought: "How can this person or this situation serve my interests?" Rarely, indeed, does she ask herself: "What can I achieve? How can I contribute to the progress of humanity? How can I work with this person and help him?"

The only thing the girl learns to be interested in is herself, her body, her beauty, her charm. The boy learns to be interested not only in himself and in girls, but in other boys, in his parents, in having fun, in reality, in life in general. Because he is more spontaneous, brought up more "loosely," he grows and develops more naturally. His intelligence develops further and he becomes more alert, more receptive to the facts of reality. Every young man has it in his mind that one day he is going to be a scientist, an engineer, an educator or a businessman, or at least that he is going to earn money, which in itself implies that he must be good at something, since the competition for money is great.

Ninety percent of the time the woman thinks about herself; only ten percent of the time does she think about reality. The man is just the opposite: he is accustomed to thinking about himself ten percent of the time, and about other things the other ninety percent. Considering this, it is not surprising that the woman, potentially the same as the man at birth, ends up blunting her intelligence. Indeed, this enables us to understand why there are so few women in the areas of science, philosophy, theology, music and the arts in general. Not only do they lack interest in such things, but the very idea of one day having to accomplish the same things the man is accustomed to thinking he must do doesn't even occur to them.

There are, of course, a few rare examples of women who developed greater consciousness, whose interest was more directly focused on reality, women who were noteworthy achievers in the manner of men. (Joan of Ark, Madame Curie, Theresa D'Avila, Agatha Christie, Melanie Klein.) I believe that the moment the woman wakes up to the fact that her universe, in which she is the goddess, is not the real universe, she will begin to rise above this and we will witness from the female ranks the appearance of great inventors, artists and composers in numbers equal to males.

When people ask me why I don't criticize the men, since so many of them are criminals, thieves, and such, my reply is this: Being the woman that I am, it humiliates me to see my sex destined to live forever in mediocrity, always in the shadow of some "great" man (envying him) or some dishonest, criminal type — a life lived in the background, typical of the person who is unwilling to step forward where her shortcomings would show and she would have to take responsibility for them.

My wish is to see my fellow females raise themselves up and do something of great merit. I want to see women recognized and remembered in history as individuals who truly helped to build the civilization of the future. At this moment I am not interested in the problems of men and what they must do to evolve.

My primary interest is to bring greater awareness of our errors, greater awareness of our pathology, so that we women can evolve and thus have something to offer in the way of help for other men and women of the universe as well as a moral base upon which to demand our rights in society.

3

Narcissism and Power

The woman, having been blessed by nature with an attractive, harmonious, beautifully-formed body, perceives from the time she is a small child that her beauty is an effective weapon. She learns early in life that she can use it to seduce, to conquer, to gain all sorts of advantages — and I am not necessarily referring to sex-related questions. For example, a very pretty little girl soon realizes that she attracts far more attention, praise and pampering from parents, relatives and friends than her little brother, whose physical appearance is less attractive; and this intensifies her vanity.

Indeed, whenever a little girl looks in the mirror and sees herself in the lovely, frilly dresses and bows and trimmings that are so becoming to her, she is aware that she is pretty. A little girl's beauty can melt the heart of the coldest, most hardhearted person, and she senses this very keenly. As she grows up, her feminine attributes undergo a gradual change. In adolescence these female characteristics begin to acquire an erotic hue that is initially fresh and innocent. Little by little the girl comes to realize that in the society in which she lives this is the only weapon she possesses that affords her greater power than men — greater, even, than that of other women sometimes. At this point, she begins to use her beauty to compete for wealth and social status.

Yet, it is precisely the woman's beautiful body that eventually entraps her in her own insanity. She becomes a prisoner of her vanity, gripped by this strange euphoria that takes command of her inner being and makes it sterile, destroying all the feeling that exists there. From this point on, happiness becomes an impossibility, for it derives from love, and only from love: love for men, love for children and other women, love for life, for the flowers and the birds, for nature and all things.

Narcissism is like a weed that overruns the intimate self, preventing flowers and fruit from flourishing there. In this sterile condition, the woman sees everything in relation to herself. She fails to perceive the world except as it relates to her own personal interests. She ponders how a certain man can serve her interests, how this or that woman can be drawn into a pact so that she will agree with her points of view and bolster her selfishness. She concerns herself with whether a particular place, car or house is appropriate as a backdrop for the romantic novel she fashions of her life, in which she is the central character.

My female friends: Only a woman can truly understand you and warn you that this attitude represents the greatest danger to your happiness, right here and now on this earth. It is the only thing — this desire to control, to dominate — that entraps us. Isn't the female's constant concern with her appearance, with whether she is thought of as pretty, elegant, intelligent and charming, a terrible thing? This obsession, this deep-rooted notion, this fear of not being perfect and worry over what others think of us, is a torment not worth the price we have to pay.

Concern over clothes, make-up, hair, jewelry and physique is a terrible prison in which the woman locks herself and into which the socio-economic system also lures her. Do you see how a gift of nature can be turned into an instrument of torture depending on the way we choose to use it?

I do not mean by this that the woman should not value the beautiful body she has been given. Much to the contrary. She should care for it with affection and respect. Beauty must be respected, preserved and enhanced. What I want to make clear here is that we must not permit our hidden desire for power and control over others to corrupt one of the most important attributes with which we have been graced. We must not use our beauty to "buy" others or to gain power. Narcissism is the wish to be superior to others through the agency of beauty — a truly insane idea. And like all forms of insanity, it brings only anguish, depression and inner torment.

The woman who perceives this will feel great relief, because she will be able to use what she possesses to better advantage. The anxiety caused by ambitious vanity generates a great deal of nervous tension which is eventually followed by stress and premature aging. This explains why highly narcissistic women age so rapidly. It also explains why wholesome women preserve a natural freshness for a comparatively longer time without benefit of cosmetic surgery, for their refreshing, youthful look emanates from their inner being.

Another aspect of the question of narcissistic attitudes, one which women usually fail to consider, is that the possibility of using the body to gain power is highly relative and extremely short-lived. In fact, no man can be controlled for very long by this artifice. The woman who uses her physical attributes to attract and marry a man with power soon realizes that her power, like all fantasy, is fleeting. The end result is nearly always unfavorable to her. When the man finds someone younger and prettier, he leaves her, alone and without money or social protection.

In addition to the inner prison that narcissism creates, a certain psychological dulling also occurs. When a woman uses her body as her principal resource, she fails to develop her intelligence and her professional capabilities to the same extent that men must if they wish to acquire power in society.

Nevertheless, the most serious element in all of this is the degree to which women are influenced by advertising in general and by the beauty industry in particular. The social and economic powers-that-be, aware of female weakness in this regard, take advantage of it to enslave them. We women are bombarded from childhood on with fanciful ideas that suggest to us that a woman's only value is her physical beauty. Books and magazine articles on how to lose weight, keep physically fit, achieve sexual fitness, etc., plus the advertisements for beauty products, wearing apparel and such, all serve to reinforce the notion that if a woman fails to dress herself in the latest styles, if she fails to use the latest products of the gigantically powerful cosmetic industry, she will be socially unacceptable, liked by no one, unable to attract a rich and influential husband, etc., etc.

The result is that women squander their entire salaries, or whatever money they manage to get from fathers or husbands, on clothing, shoes, hair and beauty care, jewelry and fur coaats —

and the entire wardrobe must be constantly renewed to keep it up to date!

Do you see how we women have become victims of this enormous industry? How we are unable to free ourselves from it because we have this inner desire to wield power through physical beauty?

Each time we purchase a pair of shoes, a dress, or even a new lipstick, we fatten the purses of the powerful. We are, in fact, taking money from our pockets and the pockets of our parents and husbands and giving it to people who already have too much, people who prevent this money from being distributed more fairly among all human beings.

I doubt very much that a woman decked out in a designer gown, mink coat and expensive shoes, with diamonds glittering on fingers, neck and ears, can feel at ease among people who do not have even one decent pair of shoes to their names, people who are cold and hungry and perhaps even unwashed, without enough money to live decently.

We don't have to go far to find the answer: people simply should not have more than they need to live decently, in dignity and beauty and comfort. Possessing more than one needs is immoral. Why do we want so many pairs of shoes if we can use only one pair at a time? By filling our closets with clothes we not only support the powerful money moguls of the fashion industry, we also help to keep millions of less fortunate human beings from having that to which they have a right: shoes on their feet.

Of course, it would solve nothing for every person who owns ten pairs of shoes to give away nine. What has to be changed is the entire economic system. Even so, if we buy fewer things from those industries which are already worth millions, we will be actively contributing to the downfall of this diabolic system of economic power, and the people's money, hoarded so voraciously by the powerful, will pass into other hands. Businesses such as small clothing and shoe industries, for example, in which the money earned goes to benefit the employees, must be organized through the initiative of the people (as, in fact, some already have been). Each dress, each pair of shoes we buy from one of these trilogical enterprises instead of from one of the large, exploitative companies is a way of furthering our freedom from the oppressive machine of the socio-economic system.

It is really very disagreeable to think that a few minds within the inner sanctums of the big multinationals decide what color dress I will have to wear next summer or what items I will have to spend my hard-earned money on to keep from feeling out of fashion, repudiated by society.

Did you ever think about how much money the fashion industry spends on advertising? Have you ever noticed that most of the ads — in *The New York Times*, for example — are directed at the female consumer, appealing directly to our feminine vanity? Imagine the amount of money they must make off of us to have such enormous investments in promotion be worthwhile! The "vultures" of economic power invest most heavily in those things that are consumed in greater quantity by the populace. If there were no market for this industry, they would soon go bankrupt — just as all of the hotels in Atlantic City would be forced to close down from one day to the next if people stopped trying to satiate their insane desire for power through gambling.

I want to assure my readers that I am in no way opposed to beauty and elegance. To the contrary; I believe that both are essential, not only to mental and physical health, but to a balanced society as well.

The fact is that the people with power, inasmuch as they keep everything for themselves, are opposed to the people in general. If we recognize that vanity is a sick attitude that brings us unhappiness, and that it is through this vanity that malevolent exploiters entrap us, then we can free ourselves from this ridiculous prison they have fabricated, this illusion that the more clothes, shoes and cosmetics we buy to enhance our mask (narcissism), the greater our power will be.

If all women resolve to let a year go by without buying any new clothes or any superfluous articles, if we make up our minds to use only those clothes that are already in our closets, then all of the power-wielding businesses that have manipulated us like dolls until now will go bankrupt. Right here and now I invite all of you women who have now gained greater awareness to act on my suggestion and save your money for a worthier purpose.

4

Women and Power

Today, after so many battles and revindications (some successful, others not), the role of the great majority of women is still played behind the scenes in society. In this book I do not intend to analyze the many injustices and barbarities perpetrated against women along the course of history. A great deal has already been written about this, compendiums, in fact, and well-written ones at that, telling in detail of the witch hunts of the Middle Ages, the wives who have been battered and murdered, job discrimination, unequal pay opportunities and a great deal more.

My purpose in this chapter is to try to alert the reader, albeit briefly, to the even more serious problem of how women contribute to the maintenance and fortification of the power structure.

Yes — this is a point I consider vitally important, since 51 percent of the world's population is female. If injustice among human beings still exists to such an extreme degree, the obvious conclusion is that we women have not done our part in bringing greater peace, health and progress to humanity. After all, women and men live side by side. It is we women who live intimately with men, who educate them from infancy to adolescence, who imbue in them the basic, perennial values of life. Whether as mothers, nursemaids or even as teachers in the schools, we have, without knowing it, contributed fundamentally to preserving today's inverted way of life.

It is we, through example and words, who teach the children to worship, serve and fear the powerful. Altogether too frequently mothers instill in their offspring the idea that fame, power and prestige lead to happiness.

Women are no different than men. To the contrary; we are all too similar in our desire for power. And unhappily, for reasons which I am not going to analyze here in greater depth, we are very often the losers in this competition.

It is the *means* that women possess to compete socially that differ from those of men. The fact that women have less physical strength limits them in this struggle in various ways, yet they have other means — which they use and perfect to the nth degree — that at times are highly effective. These include emotional blackmail, sexual dependence, apparent fragility and such.

"If you can't beat 'em, join 'em," the saying goes. And this is what women have been doing century after century. Not successful in acquiring power for themselves, they try to attach themselves to the powerful, entering into a diabolic pact with them in order to cull whatever advantage they can in the jungle-like confines of an exploitative society.

Yes, it is indeed shameful. And it is equally true that very few women have made any real attempt to modify the status quo that prevails in this world of ours. I am certain that we could have succeeded if we had ever really made a serious effort in this direction. The problem is that women think the same way men think: they want money, prestige and power. If they succeed in getting it by way of inheritance or marriage, they are satisfied. If not, then they explore other means of exploitation, similar to those men use, to get what they desire. When this, too, fails to bring about the desired result, many then develop a series of physical and mental illnesses.

It is only relatively recently that women have begun to rebel against the socio-economic control men have held over them so long. The pact that was made initially in respect to the division of "realms" (the woman inside the home, the man outside in society) has proven to be unsatisfactory, especially for the woman.

Indeed, that total state of alienation in which women chose to live, and which they obviously thought was good to begin with, has proven to be the greatest disaster for the female sex. Having thought was lost all control of the situation, women have now gradually begun to revindicate positions they had relinquished because they felt it was to their advantage to do so. They thought it was easier to live an alienated kind of life, within four walls, supported and "protected from life's problems" by a man.

From the beginning of this century to the present, scores of feminist movements have been organized, many battles waged, and innumerable protests made to combat the social injustices perpetrated against women. Gradually they have begun to acquire broader rights as citizens and as human beings. But *about* what and *for* what do women protest? From what we have found, and from the tragic results that are there for anyone to see, women want more freedom and more power, not for the purpose of bringing greater justice and dignity to human existence, but rather so that they will have the so-called "power" to do all of the unreal, psychopathological things men do.

It is obvious that women have the same right to travel freely, earn an honest living, follow the profession they choose, live with whomever they wish, and study whatever interests them. Indeed, freedom to be free, freedom to accomplish good and to be happy, is indisputably the inalienable right of every human being. But what, for the most part, have we seen to be the result of the so-called women's liberation? Women want freedom to acquire all of those insane things men want: power, wealth, prestige.

The germ of mental illness is to be found precisely in the mad, unbridled desire for power. The euphoria that comes of being able to exploit one's fellow human being, be served by others and mistreat them, of feeling "greater" than others, of controlling their lives and manipulating them as one pleases, has become the woman's desire. Not content with domestic control over children, husband, servants and the dog, women began to crave much more. Driven by inordinate ambition, modern woman reasoned: "Why must I depend on a man to get what I want? I can have all the power I want by myself."

Thus began the feminine assault upon professions that provide power and social influence. I am not saying that every women has this intention, but certainly we have to admit that the overwhelming majority waits for the opportunity to fulfill this intimate wish.

It is safe to say that women have two basic desires: to have power over one or more men through sex (narcissism and sexual-affectionate behavior); or, more recently, to develop a professional career that brings them fame, wealth and social prestige. We have emerged from a position of total social insignificance to occupy one which is even worse, for we have become active participants in the race for power.

I note with considerable sadness that we women could accomplish a great deal more good than we have thus far. In fact, many times we have either been omissive or we have acted directly to jeopardize even further the already much-compromised well-being of our fellow man.

An article that appeared in *U.S. News & World Report* (November 12, 1984), entitled "Women Expand Their Roles in Crime, Too," stated the following:

> *Arrests of women for serious offenses jumped nearly 20 percent in the last 10 years, compared with a 13.3 percent rise for men. In all, women account for about 20 percent of arrests each year. The number of women in prison — about 20,000 — shot up 147 percent in the same decade, while male inmate ranks rose 96 percent. But what is more significant is that women are more and more likely to commit property crimes, particularly fraud and embezzlement.*

This does not indicate that the female's ethical behavior has necessarily worsened; only that women's dishonesty, previously restricted to family relationships, now extends into the business world in which they participate more and more each day.

I would like to make it very clear that the notion that women are better than men, or more vulnerable or more fragile, is not really true. Such ideas are part of an extremely subtle, diabolical myth that has helped to protect women from social judgment which would be considerably beneficial to them.

In the same article, criminologist Anna Kuhl of San Jose State University remarks: "Most women are nurturers, and you can't nurture and murder at the same time." Adds sociologist Darell Steffensmeier, of Pennsylvania State University, "Most women find the character of criminal work at variance with the values of womanhood." On one hand this is undoubtedly true; yet on the other these comments show that society possesses a certain naiveté in its generalization of female behavior. Criminologist Ira

Silverman of the University of South Florida is more accurate when he says, "In the old days, if a woman was arrested and started crying, the cops might let her go. That doesn't happen much today."

In reality, most female crimes and even violence have occurred among personal relations — family, relatives and friends — because this used to be the woman's usual sphere of influence. Yet the more women rise into high-level positions, the more they cheat employers or customers, the same way they have cheated husbands, children, relatives, friends, servants and others.

According to Diane Brown, of the Greater Washington Board of Trade, in the Washington, D.C., area alone, where $500 million in goods are pilfered annually from stores, housewives account for the biggest share of arrests. (I do not refer here to women who steal to feed their starving children.) If women are the most frequent shoplifters, it follows that they will be dishonest in larger transactions as well.

Since more and more women have entered the job market (or the crime market), which was originally all masculine, they now also engage in the increasingly voracious battle for socio-economic power, as the following facts from the above-mentioned article illustrate:

> - *New York lawyer Nancy Young stole $300,000 from clients' accounts over a nine-year span*
> - *Frances Cox pleaded guilty to embezzling $48,000 from the Fairfax, Virginia, government while serving as treasurer*
> - *Mary Hudson, board chairman of Hudson Oil Company, pleaded no contest to a charge of fixing gas pumps to short-change customers*
> - *Mary Tredwell was convicted of defrauding tenants of thousands of dollars in rent money at a Washington, D.C., housing project she managed.*

The main reason women did not commit more crimes like the ones cited above is because formerly they led more or less reclusive lives centered around family and personal relationships — a fact which may indicate a greater degree of psychological equilibrium (less envy and greed).

Not rarely, however, the woman hides behind the violence of her male partner. For example, what need has the wife of a Mafia leader to kill, rob or commit any sort of violence against society when her husband already does all these things, thereby assuring her and her children the wealth and power she desires. Her position is indeed a very comfortable one.

The same holds true for any woman who attaches herself to a powerful man. She wants to take advantage of the benefits his position affords without risking herself in the outside world. Whether this type of pact is successful or not is another question entirely. Obviously it cannot bring good results, for the woman never imagines that one day she, too, will be the target of the same sort of violent and domineering acts her partner commits outside the home.

In other situations women sin through omission and alienation; that is, they close their eyes to what their fathers, husbands or sons are doing to exploit, attack or otherwise jeopardize humanity.

Behind every powerful individual, every exploiter or criminal, there is always a dishonest mother or wife to be found. The great majority of women do not teach their children that they must serve humanity through honest, constructive social participation; nor do they permit anyone else to teach them. The same holds true for the many wives who encourage their husbands to rob and exploit so that they may benefit from the fruit of these actions.

Adolescent girls are not interested in the type of boy who is honest and dedicated. Beginning in early childhood, girls admire the most aggressive boys, the ones who exhibit the greatest power — an attitude which reflects their deep disdain for reality, goodness and honesty. It is no coincidence that thousands of teenage girls faint over rock stars and artists who clearly look and act like the very devil himself.

This being the case, how can we complain of being mistreated by these same demons to whom we give all of our support and protection?

It is true that until now all of this has been occurring without women themselves being aware of it, a fact that has been to our great disadvantage in many ways, for it is precisely the "powerful" men who are most attractive to us, and who, sooner or later, crush us without mercy.

An American patient of mine, herself a psychotherapist, revealed to me that she had spent her entire youth with a book under her arm, a book which she made her new bible. Its title was *Power, Money and Prestige*. Only now, at an advanced age, has she come to realize that she was the victim of a great hoax and that happiness is to be found far from the place indicated in the book.

Women's greatest problem is that their life goal is the same as that of men. When a woman chooses a partner, a profession, or an institution to join, she is looking for a way to acquire some kind of power.

To be sure, the rich man, the man with social status, prestige, physical strength and sexual prowess, the man who has influence and social power, is automatically preferred by women. And yet it is these men who seek power, the men most interested in acquiring it, who are obviously the sickest. And of course it is these crazy, aggressive, destructive men who never spare their women.

It is also true that most nuns enter religious orders out of the same motives, since such institutions in and of themselves convey the idea that they protect those who enter there. The mother superiors of the convents have come to symbolize female despotism, envy and injustice. The story of Saint Thérèse of Lisieux is one of the most famous cases of persecution within a religious institution. This woman of extraordinary merit and goodness went through hell at the hands of her envious colleagues.

The woman who has gained a position of power can be worse than many a man. And the greater her power, the greater her tyranny. The female boss, for example, "massacres" her employees, making slaves of them and persecuting them far more than a male boss would. A patient of mine, a nurse who had worked eight-and-a-half years in the records and information department at the University of São Paulo clinical hospital, had always had female supervisors, and she recalled with horror the intrigue, favoritism and persecutive attitudes of those women. Intimidating fault-finders that they were, her supervisors took advantage of the smallest things to persecute their charges, calling them down for the way they combed their hair, the way their uniforms were starched or any lack of special deference shown to their superiors; yet questions of competence and efficiency were always relegated to secondary importance.

Today, this same person, working as a housekeeper for a married couple, two American psychiatrists, tells of the tyrannical manner in which she is treated by the woman of the house, in contrast to the man, who is always polite and considerate. The woman not only makes her get down on her hands and knees and scrub the kitchen floor every day; she keeps her until late at night, long after she is supposed to leave. On occasion the woman has insisted that she go out to the store in below-freezing temperatures, even though she did not have warm clothes. Her attention to the minutest details and frequent requests that the same task be re-done again and again demonstrate that the woman wants to take full advantage of every single minute that her "slave" is there and get all she possibly can out of the few paltry dollars she pays her for a day's work.

At the same time, the man of the house, himself a target of his wife's aggressiveness, makes a point of treating the former nurse more humanely, insisting she use his hat and gloves when necessary and often making an attempt to minimize his wife's fury toward her.

A lot of women complain that members of their sex are not chosen as often as men for supervisory positions. To a certain extent this is understandable inasmuch as so many of them, the moment they gain a position that gives them power over others, become irascible and fail to show any sense of fairness, picking on details and preventing the work from progressing smoothly.

5

The Consumer Economy is Supported by Women

Many of us are shocked by the fact that the United States spends such a large portion of its gross national product on arms. In 1983 the figure was $214.8 billion — an absurd amount of money to be allocated to destruction!

Still, if we calculate the total spent by women on superfluous things, we would be even more shocked, for the sum in dollars comes very close to that of the country's defense budget.

If you give it some thought, you will see that in most American families it is the wife who controls the household expenditures. She does what she wants with the family earnings (hers and her husband's) because she shops not only for herself, but for the children, the house, and very often for her husband as well — to say nothing of the pressure she puts on him to buy a new car, travel, purchase a new house or redecorate the old one, etc., etc.

This is why mass advertising is directed at women. Most advertisements are, in fact, carefully keyed to the female psychological make-up: the woman's narcissism (jewelry, clothes, makeup, beauty and hair care, massage); her fantasies (travel, entertainment, sex, cigarettes, alcoholic beverages, magazines); her megalomania (new house, things for the home, new car, well-dressed husband and children or boyfriend, money in the bank). And hidden behind all of this buying is a great deal of envy; for women are voracious, not just for food, but for sex and everything else that can bring them pleasure or make them feel they are better than other women (and, in many cases, better than men as well). In 1983, for example, American women spent the tidy sum of $23.8 billion on wearing apparel (not including footwear) and an additional $4.45

million on cosmetics, sums which represent only a small portion of their total expenditures.

Indeed, the consumer-related industries and the advertising experts take advantage of this characteristically feminine weakness to guarantee themselves fat profits. All of this money, which could be used to improve schools and hospitals, or for science and progress in general, is almost totally wasted on unnecessary things.

Can you imagine what progress society could make if only half of what the average woman spends on luxury items were put to use in scientific research!

If we women want to gain respect for accomplishing something of value for humanity, why not begin right here? Many of us, equating ourselves with men, complain that our salaries are not high enough. And yet a large part of the husband's earnings is spent on his wife and children. The truth of the matter is that men spend their time thinking about how to *earn* money and women about how to *spend* it. Most men work in order to bring money home, whereas a great many women do little else but think of ways to spend it.

Despite the fact that I am a woman, I have to admit that the capitalist economy is almost wholly sustained by women because women's characteristic voracity makes them the major consumers of superfluous luxury goods. In the August 8, 1984, issue of *The New York Times,* for example, I counted 32 ads directed exclusively at women with 33 others that would attract mainly the woman buyer. In contrast, only 14 ads were aimed solely at the male consumer. This in a newspaper — to say nothing of the enormous number of women's magazines whose pages are crammed with promotional appeals for articles purchased exclusively by women.

As long as the woman goes on allowing herself to be carried away by her envy and narcissism, as she has done until now, economic philosophy will be jeopardized together with all other sectors of national activity: health, education, art, agriculture, leisure and research. All will continue to be adversely affected as long as female vanity continues to be nourished.

To be sure, anyone connected with the luxury consumer goods industry will contend that their businesses provide a large number of jobs. But wouldn't it be better if such jobs were made available in the basic areas of the economy instead, such as the ones cited above? Obviously, the industry's defenders have their sights fixed on the net retail profits, which soared to the astronomical figure of $545.9 billion in 1983!

It goes without saying that women are not the least interested in frustrating their desires. That is why they allow their voracity, their megalomania, free rein and follow a lifestyle based on uncontrolled spending. When the consumer economy finally collapses altogether, not only will women no longer be able to have all they want in such unnecessary amounts; they will then also be forced to *feel* their problems, something they have thus far avoided.

6

Women and Crime

An incredible social pact exists in regard to female criminality, referred to by criminologists as "disinterest." According to Hans Göppinger, professor at the University of Tubinga, the question is not addressed with the necessary concern because of "ideological bias" and a number of pseudo-philosophic concepts.[1]

In comparison to the countless number of studies regarding male criminality, the research material available on the woman's role in crime is unbelievably sparse. Even though female criminality is far less than that of males, varying from 20 percent to 25 percent of all reported crime according to official figures, by no means can we conclude that women are less active than men in the art of causing harm to others. As I see it, the social structure has been organized in such a manner that the woman simply has less decision-making power and action. Therefore, her criminality is restricted to her particular field of social activity.

The crimes women commit are so closely linked to their sexual lives that many experts consider female psycho-biological factors such as the menstrual cycle, menopause, pregnancy, childbirth, and puberty to be the cause of female criminal behavior.

Ochman and Pollack, for example, adhering to the hypothesis presented by the French physician Legrand Du Salle in 1864, attempted to show a correlation between the robberies committed by women in the large Parisian department stores and the women's menstrual cycles.[2] This idea was refuted with considerable vehemence by Göppinger, who stated that in his opinion no authenticated proof existed that showed that female criminal acts were predominantly conditioned by biological crises.

Indeed, psycho-social factors are far more obvious causes, and in regions where the woman's active role in society is more nearly like that of the man's, as in the Southern states of the United States, the female crime rate is very close to that of males.

Although renowned criminal experts such as Pollack, Von Hentig, Reckless and Newman believe that female criminality is masked by a number of factors, it is also true that the woman benefits from the favorable opinion of the public, the courts, the police and the press, if not also from the victim himself (in crimes against family members). All sides are concerned with favoring the woman, placing her in a special category, especially when she is a person of good social standing, as Giuseppe Di Gennaro affirms.[3] In other words, women who enjoy socio-economic power tend to escape punishment for their crimes just as powerful males do.

Nevertheless, it is an extremely interesting fact that criminologists are unanimous in their opinion that the woman is *qualitatively* different from the man. Some experts even go so far as to say that the figures for female crime would be much more realistic if together with crimes such as abortion, infanticide, prostitution and shoplifting, those of slander, insult, gossip, child abuse and such were likewise reported.

Why does society consider the latter type of misdemeanor irrelevant when in reality the sins of envy, hatred, libel, intrigue and calumny are precisely the most serious of all and the ones which very often lead men to commit crimes of violence?

Despite the fact that the female lacks physical strength, she possesses a far more efficient, far more powerful weapon than any type of sharp instrument or firearm: sex.

Indeed, women — especially those in the higher social strata — often prostitute themselves inside the home as well as outside. In the opinion of Esther de Figueiredo Ferraz, renowned Brazilian lawyer and educator, seduction is the easiest road the woman can take to express her criminality,[4] and in fact it is the men themselves who facilitate this!

It is notoriously well-known that a fragile female can disarm a muscular assassin merely by seducing him. Also, delicate women not only frequently play the role of instigator or mastermind ("crime by proxy" the experts call it), but they also seem to choose crimes that offer the greatest advantage with the least risk. Because they themselves lack the courage, women "hide" behind men who do what they would like to do, leaving the responsibility and culpability for the act to the male. In his work, *Criminologie et Science Pertenciaire*, Jacques Léauté draws a distinction between political revolt and political revolution, the former being less serious, the latter of greater duration.[5] Curiously enough, he points out that while women have often played an important role in revolts, their participation in revolutions has been inconsequential — a fact that reflects the female personality. Superficial, extremely querulous, scheming and rebellious, women are far more apt to complain, to contest without clear grounds, than to propose and fight for significant social change — an undertaking that requires a more constructive type of commitment.

At the same time, we must recognize that all of the great wars and crimes have been perpetrated by men. Objectively speaking, women have never been actively engaged in wreaking any sort of destruction in the world. Yet what must be seen with all urgency is the fact that all too frequently we women have silently acquiesced to such destruction. Not rarely women adore the criminally powerful and give them affective, social and sometimes even financial support.

Women should make use of the loving, nurturing nature which is their birthright. They must bring up their children to be just and honest, and teach them to dedicate their lives to helping others. At the same time, women should restrain and, if possible, punish the men in their lives whose attitudes are dishonest and malicious. If, for example, all women denied affection and sex to dishonest men, sooner or later those men would be forced to re-examine their values.

Women possess many weapons that can be used to make goodness prevail, but very few of us actually use them. Although we have comparatively little physical strength, we are able to compensate for this lack by withholding love, care, even sex — and this can hurt a man far more than any punch in the nose. The greatest crime we commit, in my opinion, is our silent pact with the criminal type of male.

In the United States, where the woman has succeeded in securing for herself a considerable amount of social and economic power, we also find that the rate of female crime has risen significantly.[6] If women were in a position to wage war and make decisions that affect the lives of others, would they be more just, more honest, than men have been? Judging by the examples we have before us today of women in positions of power, of which Indira Gandhi, Margaret Thatcher and Golda Meir are good examples, we see that their governments are in no way more remarkable than those headed by men.

I believe, furthermore, that female psychopathology is basically the same as that of the male; only its manifestations are different. Therefore, the woman who is unaware of her psychopathological attitudes is just as dangerous to society as the alienated man.

References

1. Hans Göppinger, *Criminologia,* Spanish translation (Madrid: Rens S.A., 1975), p.439.

2. Edwin H. Sutherland and Donald R. Cressey, *Principes de Criminologie,* French translation (Paris: 1966), p.112.

3. Giuseppe Di Gennaro, "Vecchie e Nuove Ipotesi Sulla Criminalita Feminile," *Appunti di Criminologia,* (Rome: Libreria Richerche, 1970), p.185.

4. Esther de Figueiredo Ferraz, "Aspectos Típicos de Criminalidade Feminina," *Revista do Advogado* (São Paulo, Brazil), vol.1, no.1.

5. Jacques Léauté, *Criminologie et Science Penitenciaire* (Paris: Presses Universitaires de France, 1972).

6. *U.S. News & World Report,* November 12, 1984.

7

The Battle Between the Feminists

It appears to me that there are two distinct feminist factions in the United States: one with a religious base (for the most part Christian); the other, a humanistic foundation that follows an anti-theistic philosophy. Somewhere in between these two we find the more eclectic feminists, devoid of narrow-minded fanatacism, who champion any and all improvement of the female condition in life.

The first such group is marked by its moralistic outlook, especially its defense of values that are looked upon as fundamental to the traditional structure of the family, the capitalist system and institutions in general. These are the "right-wing" or reactionary feminists, whose ranks include an organization called Concerned Women for America, Inc., which has some 200,000 members thoughout the United States and whose president, Beverly La Haye, is the wife of an evangelist minister.

The other feminist faction is characterized mainly by its defense of women's personal interests as they relate to individual accomplishment of all kinds. For example, this group espouses the issues of free sex, homosexualism, abortion, and a materialistic mode of existence while at the same time disavowing any and all value systems; that is, systems based on the fundamental elements of love, motherhood, fidelity, spirituality and such. The members of this group are the extreme "leftists" of the feminist movement (they are not necessarily communists).

The most expressive group among the humanists is NOW, the National Organization for Women, with a membership of 250,000 headed by president Judith Goldsmith. Founded in 1966, NOW's most outstanding members are Betty Friedan and Gloria Steinem, known the world over as the originators of the women's lib movement.

With an annual budget of $4,550 million (1983), and having become politically active and sophisticated, they claim to have worked to gain rights for housewives, the elderly and business-women in addition to having served as intermediaries in the struggle for lesbian and homosexual rights.

A great many women consider the women's lib movement worth-while. This is borne out in an article in *U.S.A. Today* (September 30, 1983) which showed that:

> • *67% of American women agree with the objectives of the movement (according to a poll taken by* Parents *magazine in October 1983)*
> • *42% claim the movement developed their lives.*

Clearly, many improvements in the social and economic conditions of women's lives have been achieved by these feminist movements. Nevertheless, there are a number of women whose opinion seems to indicate that a certain amount of harm has been done as well. The article cites Phyllis Schlafly, who stated:

> *I think they are losers... a lot of women have been made unhappy by the women's lib movement. It teaches them to magnify their grievances, to feel mistreated and repressed.*

Certainly many women *are* mistreated and repressed, but the real cause of this problem had never been clearly defined before now. On the other hand, the philosophy of enmity and revolt preached by these feminists only serves to aggravate the unhappy situation of women because it leads them into out-and-out opposition to male friends and offspring, to society in general, and to God.

This animosity is evident, even among the feminist groups themselves. The other day, for example, a letter came into my hands signed by Says La Haye of Concerned Women of America, enjoining this country's women to form a movement against NOW. Her words: "...when she said (referring to Betty Friedan) they were going to make America a humanist nation by the year 2000, I determined then and there it will be over my dead body!" —

demonstrate clearly the intensity of her enmity toward the other group of women.

Indeed, one of the most outstanding characteristics of these groups, both humanist and reactionary, is their intense paranoia, their persecutive attitudes toward men, society, other women and even toward God. They are women who see themselves only as victims of external causes, a type of partiality that is dangerously pathological because it indicates that they take not one iota of responsibility for their problems and the difficult situation they find themselves in within society.

The lines that follow serve to exemplify the paranoid attitudes such feminists express so outspokenly:

> *We must destroy love... Love promotes vulnerability, dependence, possessiveness, susceptibility to pain, and prevents full development of woman's potential by directing all her energies outward in the interest of others.*
> (Women's Liberation, notes from the Second Year)

These movements were widely accepted all over the world during the 70's. Even among so-called Third World people, their influence made itself felt. In Brazil, for example, 1975 marked the beginning of feminist activity in that country, although their number and intensity were small at the time.

In June of the same year, the International Year of the Woman was commemorated. The data gathered at that time was unanimous in affirming that in all countries, regardless of their level of economic development, women were treated as unequal and inferior to men. Basing its decision on this information, the United Nations resolved to create the Decade of the Woman (1975-1985) so that all countries would have time to make the strongest efforts possible to overcome the obstacles that denied or limited women their full rights as citizens.

Despite the many attempts that have been made since that time, the fact remains that few concrete results have been achieved. And this leads me to believe that the real determining factors behind the situation are not being duly addressed.

One such element is the fact that the woman of today views the members of the opposite sex, and not the men and women who control the economic power, as their worst enemies.

Another primary consideration is the fact that women prefer to remain dependent on men because they think this alienated position is of advantage to them.

The magazine *Insight,* (December 15, 1986, pp.62-63) published an article by Diana West entitled "The Mystique of Female Journalists" — a report on the meeting held in Washington, D.C., involving one hundred women journalists from 39 countries: the International Women's Media Project.

Wrote West,

> *They didn't devote much of their time to exchanging news or to discussing ethics. They were very concerned about sex discrimination. At least the journalists from the U.S. were. The representatives from other countries appeared to have great difficulty in comprehending what the big problem was.*

What the author of the article tries to show is that the Americans appeared to be overly worried about combatting what they see as differences between the sexes, whereas the journalists from other countries showed greater concern over how they could develop their professional skills.

In the same article West reports:

> *Georgia Anne Geyer...concluded that men and women are irrevocably different. "Women understand issues better than men," she stated. Referring to President Reagan's Iranian arms transaction, she said, "The men who did that had no understanding of the culture of Iran."*
>
> *But her foreign panelists did not seem to agree. "I am a little fed up with the idea that if women were in power, if women could make all the stories, the world would be a pretty place," said Françoise van de Moortel of Belgium's RFTB-TV, rising to speak from the audience.*

Readers will note that the feminist ideas have not only lost much of their strength lately, but to a certain extent they are beginning to appear ridiculous as well.

Part III

A Study of Sanity

*The moment that the woman conscientizes her envy,
the moment she accepts consciousness of it, she will
leave man far behind, for she will be closer to the
angels and to God, closer to genuine truth.*
Norberto R. Keppe, *Liberation of the People*

1

After All Is Said and Done, What Is the Woman Really Like?

Many times I asked myself how women were really meant to be; that is, whether by nature the woman was originally a totally different creature from most women today.

When I tried to imagine Eve before she sinned for the first time by heeding demonic suggestion, I had a very nebulous picture of her, remembering only certain figures — highly inexpressive ones, at that — in paintings and drawings in museums and religious books. With the idea of putting together a set of characteristics that would give women today a point of reference to know themselves better, I went on to analyze the qualities exhibited by women who made their mark on history.

I found that many authors were of the opinion that the woman is totally different from the man, both physically and psychologically. Others, however, thought otherwise, seeing almost no discrepancy between the two sexes.

The Biblical image of Eve being created by God from Adam's rib gave rise to a number of beliefs, among them that: a) the woman is inferior to the man because she is merely an extension of him; and b) that the woman, having come from a rib near the man's heart, symbolizes feeling, whereas the man symbolizes reason (the head). Because of this, humanity has long considered feeling inferior to reason; that is, feeling (the woman) must be dominated by reason (the man).

After centuries of scorning the female sex, some peoples began to reformulate their ideas, often passing to the opposite extreme, as in the case of the United States, where a considerable portion of the population considers women superior to men. Theories affirming that the planet Earth is female; that God is female, not male; that matriarchal societies are more balanced that patriarchal ones; and other similar ideas have all appeared within the confines of the American feminist movements.

Nevertheless, all such conjectures have always struck me as being biased, unjust and totally unfounded. The consideration that men are by nature superior to women sounded just as dubious to me as the opposite hypothesis.

What I have been able to observe through my experience as a human being, a woman, and a psychoanalyst, is that in most societies, notably the Latin, Arab, Jewish and Oriental civilizations, the women adhere to a highly destructive philosophy of life, which they pass down from one generation to another. In fact, these women, with their deeply pathological behavior, have brought great decadence not only to themselves as individuals, but also to the societies of which they are a part, by letting themselves be considered the weaker sex.

The whole question was satisfactorily explained for me during a conversation with Dr. Keppe (the creator of Analytical Trilogy) in which he commented that he believed that God possessed both feminine and masculine qualities, and that He had divided those qualities between the man and the woman.

The woman — if she is worthy and genuine — possesses characteristics that are typically feminine. For example, being affectionate by nature, she looks after others and is attentive to detail; she beautifies life for others and satisfies their desires; she is gentle, sweet, sentimental and sensitive; and she is patient, tolerant and conciliatory — like the Creator who created the delicate butterflies, the gentle flowers with their perfume and beauty, the meek and playful baby animals, the female animals so motherly that they will sacrifice their lives in defense of their young. These same qualities which exist in him are potentially present in all women.

The man, in contrast, displays other qualities that exist in God: strength, courage, an enterprising spirit, an all-encompassing, universal mind. Thus, the union of man and woman is meant to reproduce on earth the reality that exists in the Creator.

And this will indeed occur — all the more rapidly if both become conscious of their envy. Each wants to be like the other, to enjoy

136

the advantages he or she imagines the other to have, and in doing this, they annul their individual qualities and become half animal, half demon — dissatisfied and devoid of personality.

Very often the woman sees the man as her enemy (and vice versa). From her earliest years, long before she meets her husband-to-be, the girl is taught by her mother, her aunts and her grandmothers that the man in her future is her oppressor. Because of this, society is divided from the very start. Imagine how the world will be the moment men and women, aware of this diabolic pact, become friends and complement each other!

The woman needs the qualities of the man, just as the man needs the qualities of the woman. What good is a man, alone in life, who does not even accept himself? Or a woman without affection who tries to deny her nature? By recognizing themselves as complementary beings, a woman and a man can flourish to maximum intensity and accomplish what each, alone, never before could achieve, including the discovery in themselves of totally unknown potentials. When this happens, surely there will be a far greater number of female geniuses in the history of our civilization; for as women, we possess God-like qualities which are equal in value to those the male sex possesses.

2

The Feminine Aspect of Creation

The female chromosomes are of two like factors (XX); the male chromosomes, of one female factor and one other (XY). This suggests, first, that there are essential differences between the sexes but they possess a common base, the X factor; and second, that there is an element in nature (the female factor) that is recurrent and therefore appears to be the strongest, the fundamental element in nature.

In drawing an analogy between the three persons of God, we could say that God the Father, who begot the Son, would be more feminine in essence — that is, Love; Christ the Son would be more masculine — that is, Reason; and the Holy Spirit would be the result of the union of the two: Consciousness.

What is apparent is that the woman is more closely linked to emotions and feelings (XX) than the man, who in his way of being mixes reason with his feelings (X,Y).

When a woman accepts love, her behavior is profoundly admirable, superior to that of most men; but when she denies affection, she lets herself be guided solely by base emotions such as envy, hatred and jealousy, and her behavior is then inferior to that of men, who at least preserve some element of reason.

The virtuous woman appears to be even more virtuous than the upright man. Take as an example the women who have stood behind the scientists and the artists, remaining in obscurity in the history of humankind. Such women give their men support without any wish for personal glory or power, without using the men to increase their personal prestige.

Tristão de Atayde, renowned Brazilian thinker, commented that women come closer to being either angels or devils, because they are closer to the spiritual dimension.

Andréa Salomé is an example. Her loyalty to Freud, Nietzche and others was spurred by intentions that were far different from those of the Medicis, who used Leonardo da Vinci to exhibit their social power. As da Vinci himself complained, "The Medicis created me and destroyed me,"[1] expressing his great sadness at having been the object of absolute exploitation during the Middle Ages by this Italian family of mentally unbalanced, powerful people.

In fact the majority of women who stood behind the geniuses and men of worth remained anonymous in society — like the many women who followed Jesus, offering him their work and their worldly goods.[2]

Equally interesting is the fact that after the Crucifixion, Jesus appeared first to women,[3] and a woman was the first to refer to Jesus as the Messiah,[4] which shows the women's ready acceptance of him.

And yet the Apostles refused to believe Magdalena's testimony because Judeo-Christian tradition, biased and ill-intentioned, considered women essentially inferior to men.

The fact is that the women themselves gave the men a great many reasons for thinking that way. If there were some few who stood loyally by certain renowed men, there were also many others who did what they could to sabotage them, all of which makes us believe that women like Socrates'wife, Xanthippes, outnumbered the others.

Speaking of Xanthippes, Greek mythology tells the story of Zeus, who, in his dwelling place beyond Mount Olympus, hated humanity and thus refused to give fire to man. When Prometheus stole fire from the heavens, Zeus swore vengeance. The giants rebelled and set about piling mountain upon mountain in order to reach the heavens. After waging a titanic war which convulsed the Earth and the Heavens, Zeus, victorious, punished man by creating Pandora, the woman, out of whose famous box came all of the miseries that were to afflict mankind.[5]

This mythical tale is similar to biblical tradition, which portrays Eve as the one who introduces evil to Adam and all of his descendants.

Why the woman?

If we understand woman to be the symbol of love, then we can conclude that evil entered the world through the denial of love, which is present in the inner being of the woman just as it is in the man; that is, evil entered the world through envy; and the woman, being more closely akin to feeling, manifests both love and envy more clearly.

It is a fact that the female inmates of psychiatric institutions and penitenciaries are more difficult to control than their male counterparts. Because they attack each other incessantly, the female patients and inmates require constant vigilance, making the work of nurses and guards far more difficult than with male inmates.

Isn't it for the same reason — denial of the affective element, thought of as a female quality — than men in male-oriented societies become dangerously violent and aggressive? On the other hand, isn't it also true that the societies that have achieved greater evolution are those in which the man is more ''feminine'' in his behavior; that is, in which the man more readily accepts values such as tenderness, affection, beauty and sensitivity? In Sweden, for example, where there is very little differentiation between the sexes in this sense, society is comparatively far more pacific.

The same phenomenon takes place within our organism: love is the only emotion capable of generating the proper amounts of the substances that regulate our immune system. Any disturbance in affective life generates functional disturbances in the body.

References

1. John Bartlett, *Bartlett's Familiar Quotations* (Boston: Little, Brown & Co., 1980).

2. Luke 8:1-3; Mark 15:40-41.

3. Matt. 28:1-10; John 20:1-18.

4. John 4:25-29.

5. W. Raymond Drake, *Deuses e Astronautas na Grécia e Roma Antigas.*

3

God Created Women to Be Similar to Him

Have you ever noted how ridiculous the attitude of the self-adoring woman is? How she struts along in the street like a goddess, thinking of herself as beauty personified, the perfection of Creation. How disagreeable the useless, libidinous female is, with her mind on nothing but clothes, makeup, jewelry or a man! How selfish she is in her desire to be the center of attention, pampered and praised by husband, children and friends!

In contrast, how agreeable the woman is who is a friend, always ready to help others, ready to serve her family and society as best she can — making herself useful and needed (in some cases even indispensable) for what she *does,* not simply for what she *is*.

I know that many women are ferociously opposed to the idea of their having to "serve." Indeed, they seem be allergic to the very word. But don't they realize that a person's worth comes not from what one is, only from what one does?

The human being has been graced with marvellous potential. He is endowed with affection, beauty, goodness and intelligence — qualities which are worth something only if they are put to use. In what way? If we turn inward and focus on ourselves, goodness becomes selfishness, beauty is extinguished, and affection turns into gross narcissism — much like a candle, whose flame dies out if it is turned toward itself.

God made us so like himself that we cannot act differently from the way he acts. As he said when he came to earth, we must be like him: we must serve our fellow beings as best we can and try to help even our enemies.

141

We women must stop distorting our true psychological structure and will the way we have been doing if we are to avoid the consequences that repression of affection brings: not rarely we make ourselves the Xanthippes of Creation — undesirable wives, mothers-in-law, lovers, and spinsters.

4

A Short Study of the Original Woman

According to Christian theologians, the only human being who never suffered any decadence of her original state, the only person to preserve her essence intact, was the mother of Christ. Referred to by many as the Virgin Mary, Our Lady, or Mother of God, her original name in Hebrew was Miriam.

Theological and philosophical studies carried out later say that she was born without macula (stain) on body or soul, this being why she was referred to as Immaculate. Also, because she had no original sin, she was not subject to death but was ascended to heaven by the power of God, in life — a fact which led Christians to celebrate the Ascension of the Virgin Mary annually.

Except for the few facts registered in the New Testament verses, there is very little objective information about her. This reveals that there may very well have been some sabotage done by Judeo-Christian tradition, which tends to belittle the woman and venerate the man.

However, what interests me most is to study the personality of Miriam. From what I have been able to determine, she was an extremely active woman who worked hard both in the home and outside it among her son's friends and followers.

Miriam was wholly obedient to the will of God (read the Magnificat, in which she expresses her feelings about her pregnancy, begotten by the Spirit of God) but she did not restrict her freedom (read John 2, where she asks her son, against his will, to transform the water into wine for the guests at a marriage feast). So strong was her personality and so faithful was she to the work of her son that her brilliance overshadowed that of her husband, Joseph, a relatively inexpressive figure in the history of Christianity.

On the other hand, she seems to have accepted the advice and warnings that Christ gave her when she tried to overemphasize her role and her rights as a mother, in detriment to the work he was to do here on earth. Chosen by Christ to be the mother of all human beings, she was an example of courage, initiative, vivacity and strength, for it was due to her that Christ grew to maturity, safe and sound despite all of the persecution to which he was subject.

Independent and averse to all social hypocrisy, Miriam faced with serenity the initial disbelief shown by her husband, Joseph, (and by the Jews of the time) when she announced that she was carrying a son who was not his, until he was calmed by the revelation that her child was the Christ.

Thus, having never denied affection to anyone, Miriam became the universal example of the loving, understanding, virtuous woman. Endowed with great beauty and grace, she has been the muse of an infinite number of artists. Religious tradition teaches that Miriam (Mary) is the woman who will defeat the devil (often depicted as a serpent) because she is incorruptible. But without our help, women of all races, it will be difficult for her to do this on this our planet, inhabited by so many Eves!

In reality, we should both imitate and improve Mary's example of balance and sanity, for we have many resources in our favor today — science, technology, social and philosophic development — that did not exist in her time.

5

The Woman of the Future Will Be Spiritualized

When I speak of being happy through a relationship with God, you women who are reading this probably do not have a very clear idea of what I mean by this. Repugnant thoughts surely come into your minds — as well they should!

We recall, for example, the women members of the clergy (nuns, sisters, cloistered ecclesiastics, etc.), many of them anything but examples of ideal feminine happiness. In fact, very often a woman embarks on a religious career to escape from problems that are caused by her rejection of femininity and affection. In this respect, organized religion has done us a great disservice, preaching as it has, a morbid and outdated philosophy in regard to women.

Likewise the traditional image of "wife and mother" passed on to us by our mothers and aunts is far from attractive. Nor is it encouraging to see the anguished expressions and the agitated lives of famous women such as the movie stars, actresses and successful professionals.

When I walk along the streets of New York, São Paulo, Paris, London or any other city in the world, what I see reflected in the facial expressions of the women who pass is either anguish, tension, worry or dejection; or else arrogance, vanity, competitiveness and the alienated smiles that reflect these women's shallowness. Mostly, however, I see expressions of anger, impatience and envy.

How rare it is to see a woman with a calm, happy expression — a woman at peace with herself and the world! It saddens me greatly...

At this point you are probably thinking: How can we be happy with so many difficulties in our lives?

What I wish to say is that the woman is her own worst enemy, for she is incapable of enjoying what she has in life. For example, most women spend 99 percent of their time imagining what they would like to be and have, while they fail to take advantage of what is right at hand. And if they do get what they want, they are unable to simply enjoy it. Instead, letting envy get the better of them, they begin to wonder when the happiness they are feeling is going to end, and they think up hundreds of ideas, things to worry about, just to ruin the good moments in life.

The woman makes a pact with the devil to the extent that he draws us away from the dazzling wonder of that which is from God and "dopes" us with self-illusions of being goddesses. Even though we may not be aware of it, all such self-illusion is accompanied by an enormous amount of anguish.

Happiness comes at the turning point when we relinquish the illusion that we can achieve happiness as "goddesses" steeped in envy and narcissism, and begin to live in God's happiness. The deeply envious woman is incapable of achieving happiness, for she is no longer anywhere near the joy that exists in that which is God's. Hell is living in paradise, surrounded by so much beauty, without being able to enjoy it!

In practical terms, the more envious woman always seeks situations that are inferior to her in terms of culture, quality of life, capacity for achievement and personal attributes. She prefers less attractive, less intelligent friends and primitive men who are less well off economically or spiritually. (Many men may provide social status and wealth to nourish a woman's megalomania, yet fail to provoke feelings of envy in her, for such men are poor in spirit.)

Indeed, many women go to the extreme of choosing a partner who is inferior in everything — professional standing, culture, social position, psychological equilibrium — to the point of marrying the schizophrenic, dishonest, criminal type of male because, in comparison, the woman feels superior; i.e., better, kinder, more affectionate, more balanced. When the consequences come knocking at the door, many women, unable to stand the situation, flee from it, unwilling to risk physical abuse or undergo greater suffering. They simply wanted to alleviate their envy when they chose an unbalanced partner, believing that with their goodness, their capability, they could "save" the poor fellow. Never do such women suspect that this "poor fellow" will turn on them ferociously sooner or later.

Isn't this where the idea of the well-known Pollyanna-type of female comes from? Indeed, these so-called "good" women, victims of their husband's abuse, women who suffer patiently in silence without reacting, are nothing but envious, inhuman creatures who prefer to destroy themselves, living under demonic circumstances darkened by disgrace and unhappiness. Such women would, in fact, be unable to stand a happy situation, for they would be forced to recognize that their happiness was due, not to any personal qualities or merit of their own, but to other people and to God, who provides us with everything.

Scientific experimentation shows us that everything that is truly good, beautiful and real comes from God. Therefore, living a spiritualized life means, among other things, striving to achieve the most intense and genuine happiness. Logically, such happiness can be found only:

- In good, beautiful and genuine work; for indolence and work done for the purpose of gaining power is intensely stressful and unfulfilling.
- In study and cultural pursuits; for they afford us a broad range of interesting and useful knowledge.
- In wealth and comfort; but without megalomania, envy or wastefulness, which are sources of insatisfaction.
- In good intentions; for ill will invariably works against us and is perceived by all around us.
- In love; for envy and malice bring sadness and anguish, in addition to being the ultimate cause of both physical and mental illness.
- In patience; for impatience brings irritation and malaise.
- In dedication; for inconstancy keeps us from achieving what we desire.
- In humility and willingness to admit our errors; for only thus can we correct our errors and live without tension.
- In dignity; for we must not sell ourselves cheap (in exchange for money, flattery, prestige or status), because the disrespect

this brings afterward is exceedingly painful.

- In hope; for despair leads only to inertia, destructiveness, depression and indolence.
- In charity and forgiveness; for spite poisons not only our psyche but our body as well, filling it with toxins which make us old and ugly in a short time.
- In attempting to always be pleasant to others; for the ill-humored person is inevitably alone, friendless, rejected. Indeed, who (except another ill-humored person) wants unpleasant company?
- In continual interest in useful, meaningful things; for the opposite diminishes our intelligence and curtails our perspective, making it trivial and gloomy.
- In concentration and attentiveness; for alienation and indifference make us incapable of reasoning clearly and lucidly and lead to inconsequential thoughts and feelings, therefore to an unfulfilling life.

And the most important of all:

- In love of truth, with all one's heart, all one's soul, all one's mind, placing our purely personal interests on a secondary level. If we do this, all of our affective relationships will be successful, for they depend ultimately upon the relationship we have with God.

The woman who strives to follow these premises will achieve what she desires; for only in this way will she be loved and admired the way a woman would like to be.

In short, being spiritualized means being in accord with reality, with Goodness, Beauty and Truth. It means well-balanced behavior, without extremes. The saintly person is the one who is psychologically and physically healthy; that is, the one who accepts the awareness of his or her psychopathology (errors, problems, limitations, etc.). And although we are far from this ideal, it is important for us to keep it in mind so that we can steer our behavior in this direction.

6

Paradise Lost

Having attended many patients in analysis, I noted that every human being has the memory of a lost paradise engraved on his innermost self, like a transcendental remembrance of a Shangri-La where he once lived, a situation in which he felt entirely happy and satisfied. No one can aspire to that which does not exist.

I have never known any truly sane person who felt completely satisfied with his life. A great many problems surround us, very serious problems, to which we cannot remain indifferent.

Although we do, in fact, experience moments of intense inner joy, such moments are perforce fleeting. Some external aggression, or even our own pathology (envy), soon destroys them.

There was a time when the human being was completely happy — this seems certain. But how many thousands of years ago was that? No one knows. What we do know, however, is that from the start of recorded history, the human being has exploited his fellow beings — enslaving them, attacking them, humiliating them — and he has not been happy. For as far back as we know, love has been synonymous with suffering, a fact which shows us that in the area of affection there is a very strong degree of psycho-pathology in the area of affection, mixed in with it, causing a great deal of pain.

Shangri-La, Heavenly Paradise, did in fact exist, and the proof of this lies in the nostalgic notion we have of happiness, which we seek but cannot regain. Full satisfaction left its mark on our inner being; no brainwashing can erase it totally. It is the desire and the most genuine goal of the human being, inherent in him.

It is written in the Bible that after Adam and Eve left Paradise, the man would work by the sweat of his brow and the woman

149

would bear her children in pain, for they had been tricked by the devil and wanted to be gods. Obviously, this happened to us — suffering was to become the reality of our lives.

I see that this question can now be better explained by way of the science of sociopsychopathology. Accordingly, man and woman relinquished sanity in their quest for happiness: through socio-economic power ("work") in the case of the man, and through affective life ("the bearing of children") in the case of the woman. This signifies that all human effort would be aimed at the acquisition of power and the domination of others, while the affective life of the woman would also be distorted by her desire to be adored by her loved one and by her children.

What I am trying to make clear is that we are fooling ourselves: we seek that lost happiness, that feeling of total satisfaction we once felt, and we seek it incessantly; yet we are searching for it in the wrong place, in something that will never enable us to achieve total fulfillment.

This diabolic system of life we have created does not permit us to have peace. We live in an inferno that is at once internal and external. Not only are the exploited and oppressed unhappy in our present-day socio-economic system; the powerful are unhappy as well.

And the same is true of women. It is not only the unattractive, lonely, rejected females who are unhappy; the beautiful ones, with as many suitors as they wish at their feet, are even more unhappy and unsatisfied. The powerful male together with the narcissistic female, loved by many men, are in fact the most anguished and ill content, because they, more than others, have sought their Shangri-La where it could never ever be found.

Women go from man to man, changing partners every month or so, and becoming increasingly desperate; the man craves more and more money, thinking that with just a few more thousands of dollars he will finally be happy and fulfilled. What folly! What a trap we have fallen into! In reality there will never be such a thing as the "ideal" man who makes a woman totally happy, nor will any man ever find happiness in wealth, no matter how great it may be.

What happens is that the woman, being psychologically more inverted (sicker), turns in fury against the man on whom she placed all of her hopes for happiness, blaming him for having robbed her of that happiness. Very often she will attack him fiercely with some form of aggression, moved by a desire for vengeance because she feels cheated.

The woman who is more stable, perceiving soon after she marries or begins to live with a man that she has fallen into a trap by expecting to find Eden in such a relationship, may withstand the frustration and try to develop other activities that provide her satisfaction. Nevertheless, a feeling of disappointment remains deep in her heart.

And the doubts begin: Would some other man bring me true happiness? Perhaps this one is too cold, too selfish, too inflexible, too domineering, too materialistic, too this or too that — and my true soulmate may be waiting for me in some corner of the world, hidden there: a man who understands me completely, loves me without restriction; someone who can make me feel that "lost happiness."

Yes. We know that happiness is lost somewhere; proof of it is that bitter insatisfaction is ever-present. But until we wake up to this diabolic deception and realize that no man can meet our expectations, no matter how good he may be, and that happiness does not consist in our being loved by a man and by our children, we will remain imprisoned within our own selves.

This seems to be our original sin. It is why Eve said, after eating of the fruit that was to give her the power to be like a goddess, "I was deceived." And it is why now have to renounce our fantasy if we wish to recapture happiness. We must relinquish this mistaken idea which, in fact, is what has imprisoned us until now. I'm not saying we should not love a man and our children. Much to the contrary! They are an important part of our lives. But how can we expect a human being, good as he may be, to bring us Shangri-La?

The paradise we forsook is surely more extraordinary, more magnificent than anything we can imagine: with the presence of God, in total psychological, social and ecological harmony and intense activity, replete with fulfillment in truth, beauty and goodness. Where no envy or hatred, no censorship or restriction, no sorrow or aggression, no weariness, laziness or mistrust existed: all of the riches the world has to offer enjoyed by everyone!

How, indeed, could a human being, with all of his problems, provide us all that we got from that? Even the original man, free of sin, could not!

Woman, like man, has "fallen" a long way as a result of her expectations. She relinquished her initial ideal, which was extremely rich and complex (try to imagine, if you can, what it would be like to live in Paradise at God's side), in exchange for a man (who, in addition, was also "fallen"). And the man gave up Paradise for power, which can never provide that hoped-for happiness.

The man who works solely for money and power is fated to be unhappy. The same holds true for the woman who unites herself with a man, or even thinks of doing it, to attain happiness: she will also suffer deeply, for she will be restricting herself greatly.

We must return to our original life, even though this will require effort and "sacrifice," for that is where our liberation is to be found.

Analytical Trilogy is the science that was created for this purpose — to provide the elements that will enable the human being to regain as much as he can of his lost Paradise.

The meaning of the Biblical phrase, "in sorrow you shall bring forth children," appears to refer mainly to the difficulty, the suffering, that the woman began to feel when she gave of herself, when she gave affection; for the very idea causes her great consternation and she fears that it will cause her to suffer. And only through awareness of this can we liberate ourselves.

7

The Power of Love

Women (and men, too) relate to the world through love. The feeling of affection is the foundation of everything — the true source of existence.

I am not referring to sexual love as such, for we can love a man without ever having any intimate relationship with him, just as we can go through life without ever finding anyone who awakens in us that special feeling of affection yet still feel intense love for life and for people in general.

Nevertheless, we have an inverted way of thinking, and this leads us to believe that love makes us vulnerable. Such is the case of a patient of mine, C., who believed (like most of humanity) that if she did not love a man, then she would not be affected or harmed by any problem he might have (other women, alcohol, a bad temper, etc.). In other words, she thought that as long as she avoided becoming emotionally involved with him, she could overcome any problems.

I have heard many people complain that suffering begins with love: if we don't love, we won't suffer. After all, literature, the arts and cultural tradition all confirm this idea, don't they? Even the religious community defends the premise. They believe there are two kinds of love: one, which is spiritual in its essence, is love of God and fraternal love; the other, a false, sinful love — passions which lead to perdition and suffering. One incompatible with the other.

Through trilogical scientific experimentation, we have proved just the opposite: that there is only one type of love — one true and passionate feeling that can be directed toward God, toward a man, toward our children, the family and humankind in general, all at the same time.

Human beings possess just one type of affection, and that love is human love. We are not capable of loving as an angel loves or as God loves. Yet each time that we try to prevent affection from existing or from manifesting itself, no matter who the person may be, we are in fact drying up the source of life which is meant to well out from our innermost self. The result is all kinds of problems and afflictions: fights, separation and divorce; adultery and abortion; physical, psychological and social ills; and so on.

Another question then arises: Why do we associate love with such atrocious suffering? Why doesn't a woman suffer when she is betrayed by a man she doesn't love? Why does everything that concerns the man she loves affect her differently, causing interminable conflict?

Only the person who loves is aware of his (or her) psychopathology and errors. Thus, it is through acceptance of affective life that the individual becomes able to see his envy, his hatred, his megalomania, his selfishness, and such, which manifest themselves together with affection.

The rationalistic individual ''imagines'' that he has no hatred, envy, etc., when in reality he has merely inconscientized what he feels, thus allowing his coldness and ill intentions free rein. (Many members of the clergy, for example, think that they possess a great deal of love, yet they have no compassion whatsoever.) When such a person begins to like someone, he also begins to see how envious, jealous, possessive, selfish, dominating, etc., he is. Yet he imagines that it is the feelings themselves that are bad, and that if they are repressed, he will remain sane and well-balanced. He fails to see that he has merely repressed *love* and that his pathology remains; only he himself is not aware of his insanity; for it is clear to other people.

Here we get into something that is difficult to accept, for the human being is too arrogant to admit that he must ever ''subject'' himself to anything. Love is sovereign. It is greater and more powerful than we are. Either we accept it, or we destroy ourselves. How, then, can we come to accept the idea of not having control over some aspects of our being?

This is the point at which a great deal of psychological confusion arises, and which it is highly important for us to understand fully: we see in the love object the power and the magnitude that actually pertains to love itself, and we think: "Why must I subject myself to such-and-such an individual, who has these or those difficulties (who rejects me, betrays me, is aggressive, etc.)?" We feel humiliated at being dependent on someone and having to swallow our pride and "self-love."

When we love someone it does not mean that we are submissive to that person, only that we are totally powerless in regard to the feeling of affection that exists spontaneously in us.

Any attempt to stop this feeling results in incredible suffering, both psychological and physical. It gives rise to an interminable succession of ills: anxiety, phobias, insomnia, loss of appetite, depression, despair, lack of productivity, inability to concentrate, and difficulty in relating to others, to the world in general, and even to God.

The human being sees great harm in love, and he treats the Creator himself in the same way. Indeed, the very first problem the human being experienced was related to Pure Love. We bear this inversion within us, and it causes us great pain.

A certain patient of mine had been married for twenty years to a man she loved deeply. He was a sick man, a neurotic, and he needed her affection very much. She had problems with him, but she was happy. Then one day she decided to heed her inversion and arrogance — with the support of modern psychological orientation — and begin to "take care of herself." When her husband moved to another state, she chose to remain in New York where she had friends, her psychotherapy group, her "personal interests." After some time of separation, she learned that another woman had taken her place: she had lost her husband's affection, her social and economic security, and all of the happiness she had had in her marriage.

In fact, she had thought of herself as irreplaceable; it had never occurred to her that another woman might enjoy all that had been hers and that she had rejected, especially her husband's love.

Unable to resign herself to the fact, she began to feel less anguished only when she saw how inverted her attitude had been

— that the cause of her suffering was not her husband but simply her own attitude of killing her affectionate life, something she had always done and continued to do.

There is an important factor here that must be conscientized: our entire social structure teaches us from the time we are born that we should not love. It tells us that love is synonymous with weakness; that anger and hatred are synonymous with strength, with power. Such is this inversion that it has caused a disunity between the sexes which is used by the systems that are interested in dominating and exploiting those who are weaker to further their own ends. As Machiavelli said: ''A house divided against itself cannot stand;'' ''Divide and conquer.''

If people come to see that they are victims of a process of brainwashing that incites separation and paranoia in order to further the spurious interests of those who have power, they will be able to smooth out their problems, strengthen themselves, and live in harmony. Essentially, man and woman love one another, yet everything possible is done to set one against the other.

Another important question in relation to affective life is that only that person who is willing to admit and accept his feelings (willing to feel himself) can be physically and mentally happy. I explain this in greater detail in my book *Healing Through Consciousness*.

8

A Prescription for Happiness

In addressing you, I speak as a scientist, never as a religious person. Religious fanatics have driven many people away from God by distorting his image, portraying him as a vengeful, unfeeling, primitive being who wants us to suffer so that he can achieve his purpose — a figure more devil-like than anything. I, too, feel aversion toward the mentality of the many fanatics who have caused people to feel such dislike and resentment toward the Creator.

I speak to you as psychoanalyst who for years has sought a way for women to be happier. I have never subscribed to the belief that women were actually created inferior to men, or that they need men to guide them through life or show them the path to God. If that is the way it was and is, then it is mainly the fault of our own deeply envious attitude, which eventually incapacitated us and caused us to fall from our original position, one that was surely superior to that of human beings today.

Nor did I ever agree with the idea that we are just simply meant to be unhappy, period. Or even just middlingly happy. In fact, I have always been ambitious where happiness is concerned, for I believe that it is the inalienable right of all human beings. Since childhood I have been aware of a close correlation between happiness and goodness, unselfishness and love — especially love of God. (In this sense, God can be identified with reality.)

I can say that in the past I experimented with everything that seemed that it might afford me happiness. I can even go so far as to say that I had everything any woman could want in order to be happy: a reasonable amount of intelligence and beauty, money and social status, a husband and children, admirers, sex, travel — everything. And yet only those things that were related to beauty, truth and goodness; that is, only that which was related to the Creator, brought me satisfaction.

The truth of this gradually became clearer and clearer to me. The more closely related an experience was to reality, the more intense was the happiness I felt. It gives me a very good feeling to think that many other women will be able to feel as I do, and that I can help them achieve this with my experience.

I continued to experiment scientifically, observing what the feeling of happiness was related to and at the same time trying to determine what factors caused uneasiness. I did the same with my patients. Using the process of trial and error I carried on my scientific study of happiness. This scientific-experimental approach led me to conclude that woman was born to complete God's creation, just as man was, and that only by accomplishing this can we women be happy.

A patient once asked me how we can love God if we cannot see him; that is, if we don't know exactly what he is like. I believe that our enormous envy distorts our perception very greatly, and also that we always try to compare God with something human, with the way we are, and thus fail to see him as he is. The result is that many of his manifestations go unnoticed. For example, God manifests himself through creation, and if we observe carefully all that is created, all that is real, we will come to know many of God's myriad facets.

When we look at a painting, we are able to grasp a great deal about its author; when we read a book, we can see the soul of the writer; when we observe the countenance of a child, we can also tell a lot about its father and mother.

Try to observe the things that are self-existent, those things that are original and have not been distorted or ruined by human envy. You will see incredible facets of God, subtly revealed: his good humor, in the playful little creatures such as fish, birds and insects; his beauty, in all of nature's forms; the delicacy of his feelings, in flowers, children, and small animals; his affection, reflected in music; his goodness, through the possibility of forgiveness, the possibility of recuperation for every person who returns to integrity out of the wish to be happy; his justice, which prevents the arrogant from being happy and guarantees the happiness of those who are humble of heart; his greatness and power, when we ponder the existence of billions of galaxies that he created and which he governs; his wisdom and intelligence, shown to us in the laws of physics, chemistry, biology, etc.; his multiplicity of interests and creativity, which we see in the oceans, replete with the most incredible and diverse species of living beings; his light and magnitude, reflected in the sun's rays that shine from horizon to horizon. And most important of all: our awareness, our consciousness, that shows us when we are in error and how we can correct ourselves so that we can continue on the path to development.

The examples are infinite. Try to observe this yourselves and you will see how much you come to know of God.

I believe that, although we may not be aware of it, our suffering stems precisely from our having distanced ourselves so greatly from this Being.

9

The Women of the Third Millennium

Experience and scientific observation have shown me that women, through Analytical Trilogy, can develop as much as or even more than men. In the Trilogical Residences, for example, the women have shown themselves to be honest and dedicated, careful about meeting their commitments on time, and not rarely their personal and professional performance is superior to that of the men. In the first overall evaluation, made annually in the Trilogical Residences, two thirds of those who received a passing grade were women.

If women conscientize their envy and the pact they have long sustained with the power structure; that is, if they become aware of these, they will unquestionably develop at an astonishing pace. We women have in our favor a tradition of greater obedience and dedication; greater tolerance of pain, frustration and adversity; greater patience and greater love for children and for human beings in general. Our intuitiveness and sensitivity enable us to comprehend both material and non-material questions very rapidly. Also, the fact that we have been greatly humiliated up to now has not only helped us keep our feet more firmly on the ground than men, but it has also made it less difficult for us to admit our errors than it is for men, who are accustomed to being in positions of social power and domination.

In other words, we could say that since the woman's position in society is already unfavorable, we have little if anything to lose and everything to gain by admitting our errors, past and present.

We are still making the very same mistake Eve made when she forsook God for the devil, for we adore powerful men who are no more, no less than beings fallen to a quasi-demonic state.

Those who are good friends, true friends, are rejected and not rarely humiliated by women, who use them only to nourish their vanity.

I am certain that women are going to understand what I am saying, because every woman at one time or another in her life has rejected the love of a good and honest man and has suffered for liking, without reciprocation, some aggressive, cold and arrogant man.

The greatest mistake that women in the more advanced civilizations are making is to search for happiness in the same way men do. For example, our grandmothers felt disadvantaged because their husbands had sexual freedom, kept mistresses on the side and abandoned their wives and children. In reality, those women were envious because they could not do the same, for they imagined that such conduct provided enormous pleasure. Wasn't this the path that was followed by the generations of the 60's and 70's when total promiscuity was the direction taken in the search for happiness? (A survey of 2,600 college students age 18 to 22, reported in *Forbes* magazine of February 24, 1986, showed that 31.4% thought their parent's generation was too promiscuous.)

When women realized that this was not enough to bring them the happiness they desired, they made an even worse mistake: today they battle to gain socio-economic power, decked out in a business suit and armed with a briefcase and a great deal of assertiveness. The bad results are coming at full gallop, for women are drawing farther and farther from their true essence — truth, beauty and goodness — which, in reality, is the same as that of men. The result is that today the incidence of high blood pressure, heart disease, lung cancer and other such ailments is almost the same in women as in men.

Blinded by their envy, women have failed to realize that they cannot achieve happiness by adopting "male values," for even the men have failed to find happiness with them. We could have accomplished a great deal more if we had developed ourselves in the right direction and made the men aware of their mistakes as well. But this is not what we did: in addition to having forsaken our most valuable assets, we women adopted even more highly destructive attitudes once characteristic only of men.

Betty Friedan today questions whether the women's liberation movement she began achieved its goal. Is today's woman happier than the woman of the past? It does not seem so.

The liberation of a human being, male or female, can come about only within goodness, beauty and truth. The direction which we women have taken to achieve liberation is inverted. Indeed, we fell into a trap; for freedom to do wrong, to choose evil, destructiveness, aggressiveness, infidelity or the euphoria of socio-economic power, cannot possibly bring happiness to anyone.

I am not saying that women should go on being exploited, humiliated and betrayed, or that they should not have security or an active voice. What I mean is that if we heed consciousness and keep ourselves firmly rooted in reality, we will succeed in changing the face of the earth. We will have the power and authority that adhere to the person who is dignified, generous, discerning, unselfish and honest and who fights for justice on earth. We can even take the reins of civilization in our hands if we truly want to direct it toward happiness based on goodness.

We women have been our own worst enemies because we have rejected our true power, the power which lies in our love, dedication, steadfastness, intuition, patience and sensitivity. We even fail to appreciate our greater resistance to physical illness and pain. And we have an enormous influence over our children, the men of tomorrow! We can, if we accept the consciousness of all this, force this infernal world to change into a place where we would truly enjoy living.

To accomplish this we must take an honest and profound look at our own psychopathology so that we can strengthen ourselves inwardly.

I hereby convoke all women willing to accept this difficult undertaking. I know very well, as a woman and as an analyst, how unhappy women have been up to now. And I also know how to guide them in the opposite direction, to happiness, for this is what we have accomplished through the discoveries of Analytical Trilogy.

I believe that now is the time for us to prove whether women are worthy or not. The battle against the powerful must be won by us, for we are not yet so deeply allied with such power. If in the Trilogical Residences the women were judged better than the men by two thirds, this leads us to believe that the revolution of consciousness should be realized mainly by women.

We have means, of which men do not know, to fight against the powerful. Our weapons are different from theirs, for they are neither firearms nor strong muscles. Who better than a woman to persevere in a task she sets her mind on to accomplish? We have the patience and the subtlety and invisible techniques of sabotage that no man can resist. Aren't women known to get their way by sheer perseverance?

The only problem is that we have been fighting against the wrong enemies. Instead of fighting against our fathers and our husbands, we must weaken the resistance of the powers-that-be in order to conquer them with the weapons we have, of which they are unaware. In psychological "warfare," we are the best. Now we have to use our powers against our real enemies, those who have been exploiting us and using us as objects in order to maintain their power.

In the book, *The Decay of the American People (and of the United States),* I denounced the fact that it is basically women who sustain the consumer society. It is we who, very often, pressured by mass advertising, by our voracity, by the need to quench our dissatisfaction, and also out of envy, buy things of which we have not the slightest need. Indeed, the commerce of superfluous goods is what sustains the greater part of the power market. If we become conscious of these inner problems that make us psychologically dependent consumers, we can, as a first step, initiate a huge boycott in order to break down the exploitative system until more honest enterprises are created. Then we can buy products only from businesses that belong to the people who work in them and in which the distribution of profits benefits only those people (trilogical enterprises).

It is usually we women, for instance, who buy the food, clothing, utensils and other things for the house and the family. It is up to us to stop patronizing the big multinationals and the exploitative chain stores and buy only quality articles, honestly produced by companies that belong to the people: trilogical enterprises. We can begin a program of sabotage by not buying anything unnecessary and by saving our money for better use — to strengthen trilogical initiative, for example.

By popular trilogical initiatives I mean any enterprise, work or society which upholds the principles of honesty, liberty, goodness and equality; which accepts working with consciousness of error; which is absolutely an initiative of the people; and in which profits are distributed according to individual productivity, not capital invested.

To achieve this, a period of transition will be necessary, during which new enterprises of this type, that answer to the needs of the populace, are established little by little. It will be an easy, direct way to transfer money from the hands of exploitative capitalists or governments to the working peoples.

Closing Message

To conclude, I would like to cite Betty Friedan in regard to the woman of the future:

> *Who knows what women can be when they are finally free to become themselves? Who knows what women's intelligence will contribute when it can be nourished without denying love?...*
> *The time is at hand when the voices of the feminine mystique can no longer drown out the inner voice that is driving women on to become complete.**

* John Bartlett, *Bartlett's Familiar Quotations* (Boston: Little, Brown and Co., 1980).

Bibliography

- Auerbach, Nina. *Woman and the Demon — The Life of a Victorian Myth.* Boston: Harvard University Press, 1982.

- Bruschini, Cristina. *Mulher e Trabalho — Uma Avaliação da Década da Mulher.* São Paulo: Nobel, Conselho Estadual da Condição Feminina, 1985.

- Carneiro, Sueli and Costa, Albertina G. de Oliveira. *Mulher Negra — Política Governamental e a Mulher.* São Paulo: Nobel, Conselho Estadual da Condição Feminina, 1985.

- "A Celebration of the New American Woman." *Esquire* 101, No.6 (Special Collector's Issue) June, 1984.

- Corção, Gustavo. "A Missão da Mulher." *As Fronteiras da Técnica.* Rio de Janeiro: Livraria Agir Editôra, 1952.

- Di Gennaro, Guiseppe. "Vecchie e Nuove Ipotesi Sulla Criminalita Feminile." *Appunti di Criminologia.* Rome: Libreria Richerche, 1970.

- Dowling, Colette. *Complexo de Cinderela.* São Paulo: Melhoramentos, 1986.

- Friedan, Betty. *The Second Stage.* New York: Summit Books, 1981.

- Ghougassian, Joseph P. *Toward Women — A Study of the Origins of Western Attitudes Through Greco-Roman Philosophy.* San Diego, California: Lukas & Sons Publishers, 1977.

- Göppinger, Hans. *Criminologia.* Madrid: Reus S.A., 1975.

- Hays, H.R. *O Sexo Perigoso — O Mito da Maldade Feminina.* Rio de Janeiro: Biblioteca Universal Popular, 1968.

- Hentig, Hans von. *Crime, Causes and Conditions.* New York: McGraw Hill Book Company, Inc., 1947.

• Keppe, Norberto R. *Liberation of the People — The Pathology of Power*. New York: Proton Publishing House, Inc., 1986.

—. *The Decay of the American People (and of the United States)*. São Paulo: Proton Editôra Ltda., 1985.

—. *O Reino do Homem*. 2 vols. São Paulo: Proton Editôra Ltda., 1983.

—. *Contemplação e Ação*. São Paulo: Proton Editôra Ltda., 1981.

—. *Glorification*. São Paulo: Proton Editôra Ltda., 1982.

—. *Liberation*. São Paulo: Proton Editôra Ltda., 1983.

—. *From Sigmund Freud to Viktor E. Frankl: Integral Psychoanalysis*. São Paulo: Proton Editôra Ltda., 1980.

—. *A Consciência*. São Paulo: Proton Editôra Ltda., 1977.

—. *Auto-Sentimento*. São Paulo: Proton Editôra Ltda., 1977.

—. *Trilogia*. São Paulo: Proton Editôra Ltda., 1977.

—. *Psicanálise da Sociedade*. São Paulo: Proton Editôra Ltda., 1975.

—. *Sexo e Religião*. São Paulo: Livrex, 1968.

—. *A Medicina da Alma*. São Paulo: Hemus Livraria e Editôra Ltda., 1967.

—. *Psicologia Experimental e Geral*. 2nd ed. São Paulo: Livraria Nobel Experimental, 1966.

• Kinzer, Nora Scott. *Stress and the American Woman*. New York: Anchor Press, 1979.

• Klimpel, Felicitas. *La Mujer, El Delito & La Sociedad*. Buenos Aires: Libreria El Ateneo Editorial, 1945.

• Langley, Roger and Levy, Richard C. *Mulheres Espancadas — Fenômeno Invisível*. São Paulo: Editôra Hucitec, 1980.

• Léauté, Jacques. *Criminologie et Science Penitenciaire*. Paris: Presses Universitaires de France, 1972.

• Levine, Suzanne and Lyons, Harriet. *The Decade of Women*. New York: Paragon Books, 1980.

• Lynch, John W. *Woman Wrapped in Silence*. New York: Macmillan Publishing Company, 1941.

• Metzger, Edmund. *Criminologia*. Madrid: Editorial Revista de Derecho Privado, 1942.

• Morais, Maria Lygia Quartim de. *Mulheres em Movimento — O Balanço da Década da Mulher do Ponto de Vista do Feminismo, das Religiões e da Política*. São Paulo: Nobel, Conselho Estadual da Condição Feminina, 1985.

• Neumann, Erich. *The Great Mother — An Analysis of the Archetype*. New Jersey: Princeton University Press, 1974.

• Orwell, George. *A Filha do Reverendo*. Rio de Janeiro: Editôra Nova Fronteira, 1985.

• Pollack, Otto. *The Criminality of Women*. Philadelphia: University of Pennsylvania Press, 1920.

• Pomeroy, Sarah B. *Goddesses, Whores, Wives and Slaves — Women in Classical Antiquity*. New York: Schocken Books, Inc., 1975.

• Reckless, W.C. and Newman, C.C. *Similarities in Components of Female and Male Delinquency*. Interdisciplinary Problems of Criminology, 1964.

• Rey y Arrojo, Manuel Lopez. *La Criminalidad, Un Estudio Analitico*. Madrid: Editorial Tecnos S.A., 1976.

• Rich-McCoy, Lois. *Millionaires — Self Made Women of America*. New York: Harper & Row Publishers Inc., 1978.

• Seelig, Ernst. *Traite de Criminologie*. Paris: Presses Universitaires de France, 1956.

• Shepher, Joseph and Tiger, Lionel. *Women in the Kibbutz*. New York: A Harvest Book, 1976.

• Stapleton, Rosalie M. *Woman Stuff 3*. California: R. Stapleton & Associates, 1977

• Studart, Heloneida. *Mulher Objeto de Cama e Mesa*. Rio de Janeiro: Editôra Vozes Ltda., 1974.

• Suplicy, Marta. *De Mariazinha a Maria*. Rio de Janeiro: Editôra Vozes Ltda., 1985.

• Sutherland, Edwin H. and Cressey, Donald R. *Principes de Criminologie*. Paris: 1966.

• Various authors. *Boletim No. 3*. Centro Informação Mulher: São Paulo, December 1984.

• Various authors. *Boletim No. 4*. Centro Informação Mulher: São Paulo, April 1985.

• Various authors. *Boletim No. 5*. Centro Informação Mulher: São Paulo, September 1985.

• Various authors. *Os Direitos da Mulher na França*. Rio de Janeiro: Publicações Ministério dos Direitos da Mulher, 1981.

• Verucci, Florisa and Marino, Edira. *Os Direitos da Mulher*. São Paulo: Nobel, Conselho Estadual da Condição Feminina, 1985.

• Vilar, Esther. *O Homem Domado*. Rio de Janeiro: Editôra Nórdica Ltda., 1972.

• Whitelegg, Elizabeth et al. *The Changing Experience of Women*. Oxford: Basil Blackwell, 1984.

Glossary

Action — The essence of the human being. The basis of all life is good, beautiful and truthful action. Love and thought are inner actions; health results from good action. Real action differs from agitated or destructive activity in that the latter reflects attitudes that deny real and good action. All actions designed to increase one's power are pathological. Ex.; working solely to earn money. Real action is serving other people and humanity as a whole.

Alienation — The voluntary but often unperceived attitude of detaching oneself from reality. When the individual refuses to accept consciousness, he uses many different forms of alienation: sex, power, money, hyper-activity, travel, television, alcohol, etc. Society has been organized in such a way as to alienate people from the essential things in life: love, beauty, goodness, good actions, real improvement of the human being and of society, and mainly, from the consciousness of one's errors.

Analytical Trilogy — (formerly called Integral Psychoanalysis) A new scientific theory and method created by the Brazilian psychoanalyst Norberto R. Keppe, Ph.D., which unifies the fields of science, philosophy and theology. In the individual this corresponds to the unification of feeling, thought and action which results in full consciousness. Trilogy is being applied in the areas of psychotherapy, medicine, education, economy, sociology, the arts and others, on three levels: psychological, social and spiritual.

Conscientization — An English neologism created by Norberto R. Keppe to describe the psychological process of becoming aware of reality, both external and internal.

Consciousness — Total awareness of reality (internal and external). According to Analytical Trilogy, consciousness results from the unification of love, intelligence and action, and includes awareness of right and wrong, of psychopathological attitudes, and of true reality (goodness, beauty and truth).

Emotions — The term used to designate "feelings" of love, happiness, sadness, anger, envy, etc.

Envy — Discontent and ill will over the happiness, advantages, possessions, beauty, goodness, etc., of others. From the Latin *invidere*, it means "not wanting to see" goodness, beauty and truth. Its roots lie in theomania.

Fantasy — In Analytical Trilogy always used to express the pathological use of imagination; the same as illusion or daydream. A form of alienation from reality in which the individual tries to accomplish that which is impossible.

Feelings — The only real feeling is love; envy, hate and anger are primarily attitudes against love. Sometimes used as a synonym for emotions.

Imagination — The act of forming mental images of something not present; the creation of new ideas by combining previous experiences. Healthy only when used to conceptualize good further action; pathological when used to foster ideas of grandiosity or ill intent.

Inconscientization — A neologism created by Norberto R. Keppe to describe the willful attitude of concealing, repressing or denying one's consciousness; the same as hiding from oneself something one does not wish to see.

Inner Pharmacy — A term coined by Dr. Cláudia Pacheco which refers to the natural immunological substances of the body with which Analytical Trilogy works indirectly, through psychotherapy, to cure illness.

Integral Psychoanalysis — The psychoanalytical treatment that, in contrast to traditional psychoanalysis, places the etiology of neurosis not in problems related to the libido but in the human being's desire to be like God (theomania), and in the pathology of the social structure which gives power to the most theomanic individuals. The same as Analytical Trilogy or Trilogical Psychoanalysis.

Interiorization — Different from internalization, it consists in using external reality as a mirror to understand more clearly what exists in one's inner self (feeling, thought, conscience, intuition, emotion, etc.). The principal technique used in individual trilogical analysis. The term is an English neologism created by Norberto R. Keppe.

Inversion — The process through which a person sees good in that which is evil and evil in that which is good; that is, believing that fantasy gives rise to accomplishment and that reality causes suffering; seeing laziness as pleasurable and work as sacrifice; considering God as restrictive or punishing, and the devil as liberating and the granter of pleasure; thinking that love brings suffering and that pure reason leads to equilibrium; believing that social power signifies happiness and that service to humanity implies sacrifice and inferiority.

I.S.A.T. — The International Society of Analytical Trilogy (formerly the Society of Integral Psychoanalysis), founded by Dr. Norberto R. Keppe in 1970 at the Department of Psychosomatic Medicine of the University of São Paulo, Brazil. The Society is an international non-profit scientific and cultural organization whose aim is to further research, training in, and application of the trilogical sciences.

Jealousy — Envy of a loved one.

Megalomania — Delusions of grandeur; a form of arrogance in which the person sees himself greater than he really is.

Pact — The term used in Trilogy to describe an ill-intentioned agreement, conscious or not, between two or more persons (also with spiritual beings), to hide the truth and sabotage goodness and beauty. Common among members of the same family, friends, and co-workers, it results from the belief that truth is painful and that untruth can be beneficial.

Pathological Power — The desire to be greater than others, to exploit others; an "anti-power"; the wish to prevent real power from existing among the people. Motivated by envy, some individuals wish to dominate, to control others in society, as a way of satiating their theomania (*See* Theomania). The intention of such individuals is to take happiness, freedom, money and well-being from others; not to serve others but to be served by them. Pathological power is an arrogant force used to impede life and liberty; it brings only destruction and sickness to the powerful and to society.

Powerful People — A term that applies to those sickest individuals who fight for positions of power in society and who tyrannize the people.

Psychopathology — The study of psychological illness (*pathos* = illness, suffering). Also used as a synonym for psychological illness.

Psychosociopathology — The study of psychological and social problems. Also used as a synonym for psychological and social problems.

Psychosomatic Illness — According to Analytical Trilogy all forms of illness involve a strong emotional element and can be treated solely through dialogue. Illness is caused by a breakdown of the immune system which results from the denial of consciousness.

Real Power — All real power comes from action based on that which is true, good and beautiful. Human power is linked through consciousness to the energy of God, and it manifests itself through work done to benefit humanity. Those who serve others become more powerful. Real power is based on freedom.

Reality, Real or Original — All that exists in the material and the non-material world that has not been distorted by any evil interference. All that pertains to the realm of the Creator.

Reality, Pseudo — The errors and problems created by the omission, denial or distortion of the reality found in the human being and in society.

Reality, Present — A combination of the two above; life as it is today, far different from what it was meant to be. Present reality includes illness, wars, dishonesty, neurosis, psychosis, poverty, pollution and such, together with the reality that is still intact and the good actions of balanced individuals.

Repression — The act of restraining a feeling, an attitude, an idea. Repression of love and of genuine accomplishment is the cause of all illnesses.

Somatization — The process of transforming emotional problems into organic disease. Occurs outside the awareness of the individual, who senses only the symptoms, not the emotional cause.

Spirituality — Different from religion, the relationship between man and Truth (God). In Analytical Trilogy not seen as any external act such as affiliation with a particular church or participation in formal worship.

Theomania — The megalomanic, envious wish to have god-like power; most severe in psychotic individuals and people in positions of power in society. According to Norberto R. Keppe, theomania, an extreme form of megalomania, is the underlying cause of all illness (social, mental, organic).

Psychotics often see themselves as Jesus Christ, the Holy Spirit, the Divine Essence, etc. However, theomania is present in all individuals to a greater or lesser degree.

Trilogical Enterprise — A new business model, whose objective is to resolve the basic problems of the existing economic system: each individual is a shareholder based on his productivity, not on money invested; salaries and profit distribution are based on individual productivity; capital investment is treated as a loan, not as a basis for profit distribution; everyone working in the enterprise participates in a program which helps him become aware of mistakes and attitudes that are harmful to his productivity. This proposal is different from capitalism and socialism/communism. Through this system the power of money is replaced by the value of work and accomplishment. It offers a practical solution to the economic problems of individuals and society. Since 1985, some 30 enterprises have begun to function on these principles in New York and São Paulo, Brazil.

Trilogical Psychosomatic Medicine — Medical treatment that deals only with psychological factors. Neither drugs, surgical intervention or tranquilizers are used. Healing is achieved through individual consciousness of the attitudes that cause changes in the 'inner pharmacy' (*See* Inner Pharmacy) of the individual.

Trilogical Residence — An economic alternative for living in an atmosphere of cooperation and truly human relationship, independent of traditional society. Its aim is to stimulate interest in culture and science; provide help for those who feel lonely or insecure, lack sociaL integration, or have economic difficulties of any kind; encourage unselfishness, honesty and personal growth. In short, the trilogical residence provides an environment that is favorable and effective in working with the problems and difficulties all human beings have in their lives in regard to themselves, others and society in general.

Trilogical Society — (the society of the future) A new organization of society, already established with the formation of trilogical residences and enterprises, in which people are truly free to accomplish all that is good, beautiful and truthful; in which the people, conscious of human psychopathology (envy, laziness, desire for power), do not allow the most unbalanced individuals to dominate society. Only those with equilibrium are permitted to hold positions of leadership. In the trilogical society the socio-economic structure does not prevent the people from enjoying what rightfully belongs to them: the planet and everything on it. Neither does that structure deter civilization from developing in the direction of common good. The trilogical society is based on the unification of theology, philosophy and science. It does not follow any specific religious orientation but respects the universal laws created by God.

Truth — That which is. It is absolute and the same for everyone. Truth is not relative to each individual. For example, spoiled food is not good for anyone; aggression hurts everyone; tyranny is not beneficial for anyone; love is good for everyone; oxygen is good and necessary for everyone; etc.

Index

H

Happiness, 9, 19, 20, 44, 45, 50, 75, 146, 147, 149, 150, 151, 158
Hatred, 124, 129, 156
Hentig, von, Hans, 124
Homosexualism, 85, 86
 • relationships in, 51, 72
Human being,
 • essence of, 85, 161
 • potential of, 141
Humanists, 127
Hunter College High School, 32

I

Ideal
 • in male/female relationship, 57, 74
Immune system, 140
Inconscientization, 2
Infanticide, 124
Injustice, social, 64
Insanity, 108
 • of power, 111, 114
Insatisfaction, sources of, 147
Insecurity, fear of, 35
Intellectualization, 88
International Women's Media Project, 130
International Year of the Women, 130
Intrigue, 19, 89, 90, 102, 124
Inversion (of values), 16, 47, 57, 69, 70, 155

J

Jealousy, 33
Joan of Arc, 106
John, Saint, 137, 141
Joseph (husband of Mary), 144
Judaism, 16
 • Judeo-Christian tradition, 139

K

Kant, Emmanuel, 32
Keppe, Norberto R., 2, 15, 22, 28, 41, 136, 157
Klein, Melanie, 15, 106
Kuhl, Anna, 115

L

La Haye, Beverly, 127
La Haye, Says, 128
Léauté, Jacques, 125
Liberation
 • sexual, 47
 • from social injustice, 114
 • of women, 9, 162, 164
Liberation of the People — the Pathology of Power, 22, 67
Life
 • affective, 52, 78, 140, 150, 154, 156
 • philosophy of, 25, 101, 104, 113, 136
 • quality of, 25
 • sex, 48, 49
Lincoln, Abraham, 32
Loneliness, 92, 93

X

Xanthippes, 139, 142

Y

Young, Nancy, 116

Z

Zeus, 139

Books Published by Proton Publishing House

English Translations:

- *Liberation of the People - The Pathology of Power* — Norberto R. Keppe and other authors (1986).

- *The Decay of the American People (and of the United States)* — Norberto R. Keppe and other authors (1985).

- *Liberation* — Norberto R. Keppe (1983).

- *Glorification* — Norberto R. Keppe (1982).

- *Healing Through Consciousness - Theomania: The Cause of Stress* — Cláudia B. Pacheco (1983).

- *The Origin of Earth* — Marc André Keppe (1985).

- *Algy's Secret* — Suely M. Keppe and Cristina V.R. Vasquez (1984).

- *From Sigmund Freud to Viktor E. Frankl: Integral Psychoanalysis* — various authors (1980)

- *How to Stop Crime* — various authors (1984)

- *The Worldrise* — 2nd International Congress of Analytical Trilogy — various authors (1984).

- *2nd International Symposium on Demonology* — various authors (1984).

Original Portuguese Editions:

- *Libertação do Povo — Patologia do Poder*, Norberto R. Keppe and other authors (1987).

- *A Decadência do Povo Americano (e dos Estados Unidos)*, Norberto R. Keppe and other authors(1986).

- *O Reino do Homem — Vol. I*, Norberto R. Keppe (1984).

- *O Reino do Homem — Vol II*, Norberto R. Keppe (1984).

- *Contemplação e Ação* — Norberto R. Keppe (1981).

- *A Glorificação* — Norberto R. Keppe (1981).

- *A Libertação* — Norberto R. Keppe (1979).

- *A Consciência* — Norberto R. Keppe (1978).

- *Trilogia* — Norberto R. Keppe (1977).

- *Auto Sentimento* — Norberto R. Keppe (1977).

- *Psicanálise da Sociedade — Norberto R. Keppe (1976).*

- *As Mulheres no Divã — Uma Análise da Psicopatologia Feminina* — Cláudia B. Pacheco (1987).

- *A Cura pela Consciência — Teomania e Stress* — Cláudia B. Pacheco (1983).

- *Origem da Terra* — Marc André Keppe (1984).

- *Educação Integral pela Trilogia Analítica* — Suely M. Keppe (1984).

- *Esportes: Afeto ou Agressão? — Uma Visão Revolucionária do Mundo dos Esportes* — Luis Carlos Salomão (1987).

- *Como Recuperar o Delinqüente* — various authors (1984).

- *Anais do I Congresso Internacional de Trilogia Analítica* — various authors (1983).

- *Anais do Simpósio Internacional de Demonologia* — various authors (1983).

- *Acorda Brasil - IV Congresso Internacional de Trilogia Analítica* — various authors (1985).

To Be Published in 1987:

- *Education Through Consciousness of Error* by Suely M. Keppe Simula.

II

- *The Dirty Little Tooth and The Chewing Factory* by Maria Silvia
  R. Almeida and Márcia Sgrinhelli.

To Be Published in 1988:

- *Work and Capital* by Norberto R. Keppe.

- *Liberation Des Peuples: La Pathologie du Povoir* by Norberto
  R. Keppe.

Swedish:

- *Öppna Ditt Fönster* (Open Your Eyes) — Johan Wretman and
  Cláudia B. Pacheco, Hälsokostradet (1986).

German:

- *Die Psychologie in Der Neuentstehenden Welt* — Norberto R.
  Keppe (booklet).

Italian:

- *Psicanalisi Integrale* — Norberto R. Keppe (booklet).

French:

- *Psychanalyse Integrale, La Nouvelle Psychotherapie En Formation Dans Le Nouveau Monde* — Norberto R. Keppe
  (booklet).

For more information about Analytical Trilogy (Integral Psychoanalysis) or Dr. Cláudia Bernhardt Pacheco, call or write to:

Centre of Integral Psychoanalysis (Analytical Trilogy)
6 Colville Road • London W11 2BP • England
Tel.: (01) 727-4404

ISAT - International Society of Analytical Trilogy
547 West 110th Street, 2nd floor • New York, NY 10025 • USA
Tel.: (212) 749-7441

or

313 West 100th Street #1A • New York, N.Y. 10025 • USA
(212) 864-6249

Trilogical Residence
233 Valentine Lane • Yonkers, NY 10705 • USA

or

139 Radford Street • Yonkers, NY 10705 • USA

Svenska Sällskapet för Analytisk Trilogi
Kungsholmsgatan 9, 6 tr. • 11227 Stockholm • Sweden
Tel.: (08) 50-96-09

Suomen Analyyttinen Trilogia -Yhdistys
Vironkatu 11 F • 00170 Helsinki • Finland
Tel.: (90) 633-558

SITA - Sociedade Internacional de Trilogia Analítica
Rua Cel. Bento Roma, 45 - 4°D • 1700 Lisbon • Portugal

SITA - Sociedade Internacional de Trilogia Analítica
Rua Rebouças, 3819 • 05401 São Paulo, SP • Brazil
Tel.: (011) 210-3616